Thirty-Three Days of Praise

Seeing the Good in Cancer

KARRIE MARCHBANKS

Dedication

To my daughter; my greatest accomplishment.
The light in you shines so bright, it hurts my eyes.

ACKNOWLEDGEMENTS

A cancer diagnosis doesn't just impact your life; it impacts the lives of those around you as well. I would be remiss if I didn't acknowledge all the wonderful people who contributed to my emotional, physical and spiritual wellbeing during my battle with breast cancer. So, thank you to my family, thank you to my friends, thank you to my pastor and my church family, thank you to all the doctors and caregivers. If you're reading this and your heart swells... yes, I'm talking about you! You were a blessing to me during a most difficult time and I am forever changed because of who you are. May God bless you all.

Contents

Introduction

My Story: The End

Part 1

Part 2

Part 3

My Story: The Middle

Part 1

Part 2

My Story: The Beginning

Part 1

Part 2

Part 3

My Testimony

Facts & Resources

Introduction

The end of life as I knew it. That's what my breast cancer diagnosis meant to me. At the time I didn't know to what extent or how severe but I knew my life was about to change. The definition of what it meant to be me had just been rewritten and no one, least of all me, could have predicted the emotional, physical, financial and spiritual upheaval a cancer diagnosis generates. Cancer is a pernicious viper, it slithers its way into your life unannounced, ready to strike at the worst possible moment and there's seemingly nothing you can do about it.

Before my diagnosis, I was living my life without a care in the world! Basking in the accolades of my first book; *Sweet Tea and Cornbread,* proudly watching my daughter maneuver her way up the corporate ladder, happy to have found a new church home and more fit and healthy than I had been in years. Life couldn't get any better! And so, it got worse. Seemingly out of nowhere I was blindsided with a breast cancer diagnosis and everything that was good and perfect in my world was turned upside down and I was left shaken and lost from the unexpected turn of events. It's times like these when your faith is tested, when you all of the sudden get religious and you and Jesus are on a first name basis. When you're diagnosed with breast cancer, just hearing the words and your name in the same sentence, is enough to send you over the edge. Survival becomes instinctual and surrender is not an option.

It's not easy to see the good in something that by its very nature tends to be so devastating. But if you can take yourself out of the equation, step back and see the big picture; it's your perspective about what you're going through that changes everything. An egg boiled in water will harden, but a potato boiled in that same water will soften. As Christians, it's up to us to decide whether we will harden our hearts and lose faith when we are thrust into the fire of testing or if we will we soften our hearts and faithfully believe that God is in control and that no weapon formed against us shall prosper.

Now that I am safely on the other side of my battle with breast cancer I have learned that with every challenge life throws at you comes the opportunity to be blessed. *Thirty-Three Days of Praise* is more than just a story of survival. It is a story of challenge and opportunity. A story of God's love and faithfulness and a story of victory! As you accompany me on this journey you will witness the end of my life as I knew it, and the beginning of my life as a servant of God. You'll understand through my testimony that when you unlock the most powerful weapon we as Christians' have, you can take the worst thing to ever touch your life, and turn it into a blessing that will change your life forever! *Thirty-Three Days of Praise* is a story about how I was able to use that weapon to see the good in cancer and after reading this book I pray you will not only be able to see the good in the challenges you're faced with, but in so much more. God bless you!

My Story: The End

Part 1

I remember like it was yesterday. I had decided to eat my lunch in the car and had just popped in disk number fifty-two of my audio bible when the phone rang. I glanced at the screen, annoyed by the caller who had the audacity to interrupt my quiet time. I didn't recognize the number and hesitated to take the call, but this time, instead of letting it go to voicemail, I pressed answer and took the call.

"Hi, Ms. Marchbanks! This is Sherri from Ballantyne Radiology. I'm calling to let you know that we need to have you come back in to be re-examined. There's no need to worry," she said. "This is just standard procedure." She went on to explain, "The images we took show a change from last year, so the doctor has ordered another mammogram just as a precaution."

In all my life I had never received a call-back from a mammogram appointment and my thoughts quickly rushed toward judgment. *Somebody messed up and they're trying to cover their tracks, that's all. They better not charge me for a second visit!* The woman continued on in the same cheerful voice.

"We would like to schedule your appointment at the Breast Center in South Park so you won't have to wait for the results. A doctor will be available to go over the findings with you immediately following the exam."

Still annoyed at the interruption, I quickly settled on a date for the follow-up, said goodbye and re-adjusted the volume of the radio. I took a bite of my tuna salad sandwich and laughed at the sound of Denzel Washington's voice speaking the ancient biblical words of King Solomon with his distinct New York accent. *Why would they call you back if everything was okay? What if they found something?* From out of nowhere the enemy's malicious thoughts crept into my mind, trying to distract me. I focused my attention back to the Word. *You say you don't fear death, that you're excited about going to heaven. Are you sure about that?* I shook the evil thoughts from my head and confronted the enemy right there in the car.

"Yes, I am! No weapon formed against me shall prosper! God loves me! He has plans for me, so be gone! I rebuke you in the name of Jesus!" And just as quickly as the negative thoughts arrived, they were gone. I have since imagined that on that day, at that very moment, God and the angels were looking down from heaven, giving each other high fives and shouting, "You go girl!"

Fast forward, two weeks later. I arrived at the Breast Center fifteen minutes early. With time to spare, I closed my eyes and said a quick prayer. *Lord, thank you for the blessings you have given me and those I have yet to see. I know you are with me today, and I trust you with my life. Amen. Let's do this!* I took a deep breath and exited the car. The moment I walked through the doors I knew I was not in a typical mammogram office. What was my first clue? The number of couples in the waiting area. I scanned the room as I walked toward the reception desk and was stunned by the sight. The significance of the appointment became perfectly clear and my stomach fluttered.

"Karrie Marchbanks, here to see Dr. Raine," I said to the receptionist. She looked up from her papers and smiled as she asked for my insurance card. She asked all the usual questions: "Do you still live at this address? Is this your correct phone number? Have there been any changes with your insurance?" And then told me to have a seat and the nurse would call me back as soon as possible.

I took a seat in a chair against the wall and surveyed the crowd. There were so many couples in the room that it made me question why I hadn't thought to bring someone with me. I was the only single person in the entire waiting room, and for a second I felt completely alone. *They didn't tell me to bring someone with me. Was I going to need someone?* Just then, the Lord showed me His Glory and I looked to the empty seat next to me. *I'm not alone; God is sitting right here, next to me.* I smiled and a peace washed over my body as I began thanking Him for always standing by my side. *Thank you, Lord! Thank you for your comfort, thank you for your peace, thank you for the blessings you have given me and those I have yet to see. You are Lord God Almighty and you are with me! Hallelujah!*

"Ms. Marchbanks?" the nurse called as she came through the door. The sound of her voice startled me out of my prayer. I opened my eyes, smiled toward the empty seat next to me and followed her back to the changing room.

"Undress from the waist up and put on the exam smock with the opening to the front. Just open the door when you're ready and I'll take you to back."

I didn't have to wait long for her to return and lead me down a short hallway to the x-ray room where she would perform the mammogram. She explained what her role was to be during this visit and what would happen after the pictures had been taken. She told me how great Dr. Raine was and said she thought I would really like her. *Ah, here we go. I hate this machine … just another way to torture women in the name of preventive medicine.* The nurse struggled to stretch what little bit of breast tissue I had onto the platform, and I struggled not to elbow her in the face because she was hurting me! She took pictures every which way but inside out, then finally released me from the vise grip of the machine and led me back to the changing room to wait for the doctor. I dressed, sat down in a nearby chair and prayed for a positive outcome.

Dr. Raine was a tiny woman. She had dark brown hair that fell to her shoulders, brown eyes and very petite, very cold hands. She reminded me of Sally Field. Her smile was warm as she shook my hand and asked how I was doing.

"I've been better," I said with a nervous laugh. She sympathized with me and proceeded to explain the results of the mammogram.

"The images we just took confirm that there are four areas in your right breast that could be cancerous, so I am recommending we do a biopsy as soon as possible to rule it out." She went on to explain why the x-rays were inconclusive and why she felt the need for further action.

Questions were racing though my mind so fast I couldn't hold on to one of them long enough to verbalize it, so I sat there, in silence, until she was finished.

"Do you have any questions?" she asked.

"No." I lied, while shaking my head in disbelief. Doctor Raine stood up to exit the room. She handed me a pamphlet explaining what we had just talked about and then reached into her pocket and pulled out her card.

"Feel free to call me if you think of anything later; they will schedule the biopsy appointment up front." She smiled. I said, "Thank you," and then we shook hands and she left the room. The nurse hesitated for a second before leaving, which was just enough time for me to find my voice.

"I want to see it."

"See what?" she asked.

I looked up until our eyes met. "I want to see it. I want to see what she's talking about. I need to know what I'm praying against." The look in her eyes told me she was puzzled by my request, but the smile on her face assured me she understood my need.

"Let's go," she said, and together we walked back to the x-ray room where she pulled up the test results on the computer. My eyes immediately zeroed in on the four, white, oblong spots on the monitor. I looked to the name at the top left hand side of the screen. It read, Karrie Marchbanks, then back to the spots and back to the name again. I struggled with the reality that the image on the screen was actually of my breast. The nurse was able to show me the results of my mammogram from last year versus the results from this year and explained again why doctor Raine thought the biopsy was the next course of action. She watched me, waiting for my reaction.

"Okay," I said, and turned to leave the room with the image of the four white spots imprinted on my brain forever. I walked to the waiting area in a daze, almost forgetting to stop at the reception desk. I felt vulnerable, exposed, like everyone sitting there could now see I had spots in my breast. Silly, huh? Or, perhaps, just normal. I had just received news that could alter the very biology of my body, news that could change my life forever and I was scared.

The appointment for the biopsy was scheduled at the main hospital. *Funny,* I thought to myself, *I've lived in Charlotte for thirteen years and have never been to the hospital, until now.* The axis of the world tilted ever so slightly and I found myself feeling dizzy; a feeling of heaviness in my chest made it hard to breathe. It felt like every cell in my body was going to explode and make a fine mess if I didn't get out of that building, so I made my way as quickly as I could toward the parking lot.

"There's no way! There's no way!" I shouted out loud as I took my seat in the car, my mind chaotic from the stampede of random thoughts that were now forcing their way into my head. I drove as quickly as I could through the traffic of the busy streets, trying to get as far away from that office as possible. I just wanted to go home! I needed to be home where I could lie down on the floor, turn on my worship music and pray to God to fix this! But it seemed at every turn the enemy was on to my plan, literally placing road blocks in my path. He seemed determined to preempt the barrage of prayers this new found prayer warrior was about to unleash against him and the four white spots that dared to threaten my very existence.

By the time I got home I was so worked up. I had

barely walked through the door when I let out a cry so loud it shook me to my core and reverberated through the empty rooms. I ran up the stairs to my bedroom and fell to the floor. I prayed and cried and then prayed some more, trying to think of all the things I had learned from my Pastor, Pastor John, because now, I was on a mission!

Determined to use my faith to make the spots disappear, I got olive oil, anointed my hands and prayed over my breast. I spoke words of life over my situation and praised God for the healing that was already taking place. I even closed my eyes and visualized myself going in for the biopsy and the doctors being dumfounded by the fact that the spots were no longer there. I had complete confidence that with the Lord's help I could do this.

As I reflected back through previous sermons and bible study classes, it didn't take long for me to realize that the months leading up to today had prepared me for this very moment. God had equipped me to know that it is praise that quiets the mind and brings peace during times of despair! And it is the name of Jesus that strengthens and heals! And it is the Holy Spirit who anoints me and seals the victory! And…and; I wasn't afraid anymore.

I received a text message from Pastor John that evening. He said he was just checking on me and asked how I was doing. He didn't have a clue what I was going through at the time, *or* did he? I simply replied back with, "*I'll let you know in a few days, LOL!*" and left it at that.

My Story: The End

Part 2

When the day finally arrived for the biopsy, I was fired up and ready to go! I woke up that morning, showered, even shaved my legs because today I had something to prove and I felt like struttin' my stuff for the whole world to see. I put together an outfit that screamed, *full of life and cancer free*, then quickly curled my hair and applied my makeup. I couldn't wait to see the look on Dr. Raine's face when she realized the white spots were gone! I had even rehearsed what I was going to tell her, how I went home, prayed, anointed myself with oil and was healed by the blood of Jesus! *What a great day this is going to be! My testimony might even bring some people to Jesus! Glory to God!*

I followed my navigation system's instructions down highway seventy-seven to the main campus of Carolina's Medical Center. Traffic near the hospital was crazy and in all the madness I missed my turn which sent me on an impromptu tour of the hospital's campus; boy was it big! I weaved my way up and down a maze of one way streets before finally reaching my destination. The hospital was a medical village of sorts, complete with restaurants, police and aerial transportation. It is home to the only Level One Trauma Center in the southern region of the state, Levine Children's Hospital and the Levine Cancer Institute, and today it is the location of the outpatient surgery center where I will be undergoing a biopsy to determine whether or not I have breast cancer.

I can count the number of times I've been admitted to a hospital on two fingers — to be born and to give birth — so this was all new to me. I parked my car in the nearby deck and entered the facility on the second floor. A short walk took me to a set of stairs that lead to the lobby down below. There was a concierge desk in the center of the main level, so I walked in that direction.

"Can I help you find some*ting* ma'am?" the woman behind the desk asked with a rich, Caribbean accent.

"I'm here to see Dr. Raine in outpatient surgery."

"But of course!" She smiled and pointed in the direction of the elevator. "Take the elevator down to the fourth floor and exit to your left. Look for the door with the big pink ribbon on it. They'll take care of you there. Oh, and if you need some*ting* to eat, there's a Chick-fil-A on the fifth floor."

"Thank you," I said, and hurried to catch the next elevator. Once inside I pushed buttons four and five and rode the short distance down to the fifth floor. The elevator doors opened and the smell of chicken and waffle fries made my empty pre-op stomach tighten with a growl. I poked my head out for a quick look around, and sure enough, there was a full-service restaurant, packed with people and operating at full tilt. I pulled back just as the doors started to close and shook my head. *When did they start putting fast food chains in hospitals?*

The concierge was right on point when she told me to look for the door with the big pink ribbon. There it was to the right of the waiting area for all to see. I felt a little unsettled as I approached the door — not because of the biopsy; God had that covered, but that BIG pink ribbon! It screamed BREAST CANCER to me and I felt like if I walked through the door I would be claiming the diagnosis. I froze for a second; my hand stretched outward reaching toward the doorknob. I could feel the eyes of the people in the waiting room on my back and suddenly had the urge to turn around and shout to the room, *"Nothing to see here folks! I don't have breast cancer; I'm just here for a biopsy. Go back to reading your magazines. Everything is under control!"* I chose, instead, to take a deep breath and walk through the door. With the click of the lock behind me, I exhaled and took several determined steps toward the reception desk.

I didn't have time to pray or reflect this time; before I could sit down and get comfortable the nurse was calling me to the back. She led me to a changing room where I donned the typical blue paper smock, opening to the front, and waited for her to return. Nurse one — I call her that because I had a team of caregivers that day — led me to the surgery room. As we walked she told me her sole duty was to make sure I was comfortable and had everything I needed, which at the time I thought was very odd. We entered a room that had what looked like a massage table in the center of it. Machines, computers and medical paraphernalia lined the perimeter. *Why would they put the hole for your face in the center of the table like that?* As if nurse one were reading my mind, she began instructing me on the proper way to lay on the table, which was face down, surgery boob through the hole, arms at my sides, and head turned to the left or right, whichever was most comfortable. *Oh! Boob through the hole! Got it!*

She went on to say, "Make sure you're in a comfortable position because once I map the surgical area you must hold perfectly still. No movement at all."

I climbed onto the table, removed my smock, positioned my right breast perfectly into the hole, made one last adjustment and announced that I was ready. The nurse covered me with a warm blanket and proceeded to map the area of my breast where the biopsy would be taken.

In the distance I heard footsteps approaching and then a voice say, "Hi, Ms. Marchbanks. Looks like we're ready to get started." It was Dr. Raine and nurse number two. "This procedure won't take long and you shouldn't feel any pain. I'll be using a core biopsy needle to make the extraction and we will continue to administer the anesthetic during the biopsy to keep you as comfortable as possible. It is important for us to know exactly where the parameters of the masses are, should you need to undergo surgery, so I may have to take more than one biopsy. Once I've collected all the samples, they will go to the lab and I should have the results for you in a couple of days. Do you have any questions before we get started?"

"No," I answered.

"Are you comfortable?" she asked.

"Yes," I replied and began to pray. *Dear Lord, you are a mighty God and I thank you for the healing that has already taken place. Please guide Dr. Raine's hands. In Jesus' name I pray, Amen.*

The reason for the inverted surgical technique became apparent as the table started to rise. By dangling the breast through the hole they were able to stabilize the area and ensure a more accurate biopsy. Dr. Raine positioned herself under me and proceeded to inject my right breast with anesthetic. The liquid burned as it entered my body; I felt it traveling through the tissues, working its way in with cold precision. After one more injection Dr. Raine began mapping the extraction point with coordinates obtained from a nearby computer.

"Ok, everything looks good," she announced. "I'm going to start the biopsy." She made an incision with a scalpel just large enough for the needle to go through, and then slid her stool back to grab an instrument handed to her by nurse two. I glanced up just in time to see the "needle" she had referred to. To me it looked more like a meat thermometer than a needle. *Is she really going to stick me with that?* The answer was yes, and doctor Raine inserted the metal tube into my breast. Fortunately, the anesthetic was doing its job and the only sensation I experienced was heavy pressure. Nurse one, my designated comfort coach, stood by my side and gently rubbed my back, offering words of encouragement throughout the procedure.

"You're doing fine," she would say in a calm, soothing voice. This seemingly insignificant task spoke volumes to the type of care and treatment that went on behind the door with the big pink ribbon. It was in that moment that I came to realize that the pink ribbon stood for more than just breast cancer; it also stood for dignity and respect, sisterhood and well-being, and represented a place where women cared for women … a place where you felt safe and in good hands. I had come there with the intention of being a blessing to them with my testimony of healing, but their compassion was just as much a blessing to me.

As I lay on the table, meat thermometer poking around in my breast, I became aware that I had a clear view of a computer monitor just behind Dr. Raine. There was an image on the computer screen that looked just like the image taken at the breast center; four white, oblong spots shown clear as day. I was just about to rationalize it all away when out of nowhere appears something that looks like the biopsy needle sliding in from the bottom of the screen. I watched as the shaft made its way to the white spots, engulfed them and then exit as quickly as it appeared. *That's me! That's me on the screen!* My heart sank with the affirmation that the spots were still inside my body. *How can that be? I prayed, I anointed myself with oil, I asked God for healing! Why are the spots still there?* Nurse one's hand stopped rubbing my back and she leaned over the table to look at my face.

"Are you okay?" she asked. Was I? I didn't know. My insides were screaming *NO*, but my mouth had already formed the word "Yes," so that's what I said.

Dr. Raine took one more sample, handed it to nurse two and began stitching me up. The entire process from beginning to end took mere minutes and I was off the table and on my way back to the changing room with nurse one.

"Go ahead and get dressed and I'll be right back." When she returned she was carrying a small, flat icepack.

"Place this inside your bra over the surgical site; it will help reduce the swelling and or bruising and provide some pain relief once the anesthetic wears off." she said. She also handed me a sheet of paper which outlined a list of post-op do's and don'ts and told me Dr. Raine would be in shortly. She appeared at the curtain seconds later.

"How are you feeling?"

"I feel great!" I replied, with probably too much enthusiasm.

She smiled. "Don't hesitate to call the number on the paper if you have any questions or any concerns. I'll call you as soon as the results are in."

And that was it. I walked out the door with the big pink ribbon, ice pack tucked discretely inside my bra and my head held high in complete defiance of those white spots. *It's okay, it's going to be okay. Everything's going to be okay. I do not have breast cancer!*

I waited for what felt like hours for the elevator to reach my floor. When it finally arrived there was a group of people huddled around me waiting to get inside. I entered and moved toward the button side of the elevator in hopes that no one would notice the gauze wrapped ice pack now peeking out from inside my v-necked shirt. *Why did I wear this stupid shirt? Everyone can see this stupid ice pack!* When the doors opened on the fifth floor, I wasn't as impressed by the restaurant as I had been before. In fact, I didn't even notice the smell of food. I was too busy being irritated by yet another delay. *Where are all these stupid people coming from? I just want to get out of here, please!* There had been a definite change in my mood since I left the house skipping through the daisies that morning. God had some *splainin'* to do and He and I were going to have a long talk if I could ever get out of this stupid elevator and into my stupid car!

As the doors opened on the main level I pushed past

everyone as quickly as I could and rushed toward the stairs. I would have taken them two-by-two had I not been afraid of losing the icepack; Lord knows I didn't want to draw any more attention to myself! Eyes downward, mind elsewhere, I almost bumped into a man coming through the door from the parking deck. He was taller than me, which is rare, and had the most beautiful blue-green eyes.

"I'm sorry, excuse me," he said with a smile. "Um, could you tell me if this is the building for one-day surgery? I'm completely lost."

Now, any other day, any other time, my flirt instincts would have kicked in and I would have flashed a devastatingly beautiful smile his way and offered up my sunny disposition while simultaneously showing him the lack of ring on my left hand. But today, he was lucky I responded at all! *Can't you see I'm in a hurry?* Trying not to sound rude, I answered his question with a polite, albeit curt, "Yea, take the stairs down to the first floor. Can't miss it," and pushed past him, determined to reach my destination.

When I finally made it to my car I just sat there. I didn't cry, I didn't shout, I wasn't even mad at God; I was scared. I was afraid my faith in the healing power of Jesus wasn't strong enough or that I had missed a step or something when I anointed myself with oil. *What did I do wrong?* My mind immediately went to a story Pastor John had told the church one Sunday. In his sermon he said, "The same power Jesus Christ has, you have through the blood of His sacrifice." And he had the whole congregation laughing when he told us that he should be "slipping on oil by the time he walks into a hospital room," because we've already laid hands on the sick. So, why was I not healed? Why were the spots still there? I had prayed for a miracle; was I not deserving of one? The questions attacked my spirit all the way home until I was convinced the only thing left for me to do was to pray harder. *Ok, so the spots are still there. So what! The victory will come when the test results come back negative. My God is Jehovah Rapha my healer and I am covered by the blood of Jesus! Hallelujah!*

That afternoon as I continued the ice treatments, I prayed to God and let Him know I still believed. *Dear God, you are my Lord and Savior. You are the beginning and the end. I praise your Holy name! I am nothing without you, Lord. I have nothing without you. You are Jehovah Nissi, my provider. Thank you for the food I ate today, the clothes I'm wearing, the job that pays the bills, the car that takes me from place to place, and the roof over my head. You are Jehovah Rapha, my healer and I am believing you today for a miracle, Lord. I pray that the test results will come back negative because you are a mighty God! The enemy is a liar! No weapon formed against me shall prosper. Glory to God! Thank you, Lord! In Jesus' name I pray, Amen! Hallelujah!* And so the waiting game began.

My Story: The End

Part 3

I'm still getting used to the fact that my baby girl is now a grown woman. I have loved every minute of being her mother and while there is a certain satisfaction at watching my best work fulfilling her destiny, I miss her presence at home. It's been a couple of months since she accepted the job promotion and was transferred out of state — a big change for both of us. Fortunately, she's close enough for me to get to her by car in an emergency, but far enough away for me to think twice about popping in for a visit. I haven't seen her since I helped her move into her new apartment and I'm looking forward to spending time with her and my grand-dog, Remy.

The drive from Charlotte to Savannah is about three and a half hours. It's an easy drive and not a lot of traffic, but boring as heck! Interstate ninety-five is a tree-lined tunnel of asphalt with intermittent breaks in the foliage just wide enough for the crafty undercover state trooper to make his lair. It's Thursday, three days after my biopsy and I'm looking forward to getting out of town for a long weekend. The car is packed; my stack of carefully selected road music sits conveniently on the front passenger side seat along with an apple, some trail mix and a bottle of water; I'm ready to go. *I wish they would go ahead and call me with the results of the biopsy! All this waiting is killing me!*

I would travel uninterrupted all the way to Orangeburg, South Carolina before the call came. I turned down the music and touched the Bluetooth in my ear to answer the phone.

"Hello, Karrie?" The sound of Dr. Raine's voice made my stomach ache. "I've got the results from the biopsy. Is this a good time?"

As good a time as any. "Hi, Dr. Raine. Yes, go ahead. I'm just driving down the road."

"Oh … Oh, okay." She sounded a little nervous about the fact that I was driving. "Well, the biopsy results show that the cells we extracted are malignant, which means they are cancerous. But the good news is we caught it early and it is a form of cancer that is highly treatable… Are you there?"

I don't think I breathed a single breath of air after the word "cancerous," and struggled to take a breath even now in order to respond to her question. "Yes, I'm here."

She went on to explain what type of cancer it was, where it was located and the recommended course of treatment.

"I'm going to send the results over to your primary

care physician and she'll take it from there. Are you okay? Do you have any questions?"

If I did I couldn't think of them now; and as far as being okay … in what sense? I chose my words carefully because I knew that whatever sprang forth from my mouth at this moment would either be intercepted by the enemy *or* covered by God's grace. I chose to speak life into my current circumstances.

"I'm just glad you called me today! Now I don't have to worry about it over the weekend. I'm on my way to Savannah for some fun in the sun with my daughter. I'll call Dr. Weston on Monday when I get back."

"Wow, Karrie, I love your attitude about this! You're exactly right; don't worry and enjoy your weekend with your daughter. I'm sure Dr. Weston will be in touch with you before Monday. She will want you to schedule an appointment with a surgical oncologist as soon as possible."

"Great! Thanks, Dr. Raine. Have a wonderful weekend."

"You're welcome; goodbye."

"Bye!"

Tears welled up in my eyes as the conversation with Dr. Raine looped over and over again in my mind. *She was talking about me, right? She said I had cancer, right? She said I have cancer!* The knot in my stomach tightened and for a second I thought I might throw up. My mind was overwhelmed with questions. *How could this happen? What did I do to cause this to happen? Was it something in my diet? Was I not exercising enough? Was it the birth control pills I was taking to reduce the side effects of perimenopause?* I had no answers, only questions, and the more I thought about it the more it made me sick. Then I got angry! *I'm in the best shape of my life! I eat healthy, exercise, drink nothing but water! Why me? I wrote a book about how to live a healthier lifestyle for Pete's sake! I don't smoke, don't drink; how could this happen to me?* I went through the Five Stages of Grief in the span of about ten minutes. *Stop it! Stop it right now! You are not going to do this! You're better than this; you're a child of God! Do not give this thing anymore of your power. Enough!* I can tell you without a shadow of a doubt that if it were not for my faith in God, Jesus and the Holy Spirit, I would have been a complete mess by the time I reached Savannah, but once the acceptance stage finally kicked in I knew what I had to do — pray ... so I did.

The phone rang in my ear and made me jump! I quickly refocused and grabbed my cell to see who was calling. It was my daughter. I cleared my throat, put a smile on my face and pressed the Bluetooth button to answer the call.

"Hi, Lovie! Whatcha doin'?"

"Where you at?" she asked, her voice sounding like a teenager.

"About twenty miles from ninety-five. Why, what's up?"

"Just checking. I get off at five, but you'll probably beat me to the apartment as slow as traffic moves in this town."

I laughed out loud. "Patience, Lovie. Don't be in such a rush! I can't wait to see you."

"Me, too!" she said, and I could hear the smile nestled in the warmth of her voice.

Tell her, tell her! "Hey, the doctor called with the results of my biopsy."

"Okay?" She responded with trepidation.

The words that came out of my mouth next were the hardest words I've ever had to say. My mouth went dry and the words stumbled out as if I were speaking English for the very first time.

"She said I have breast cancer." The words tasted foreign in my mouth and I desperately wanted to choke them back and swallow them whole in an attempt to undo that which was already done. "But we caught it early, so there's nothing to worry about. I'm not worried, so don't you be worried. We'll talk about it more when I get there. Okay?"

"Okay," she replied hesitantly.

"Seriously, baby, there's no need to worry. I'm going to be fine, okay?" I wanted to reach out and hold her in my arms.

"Okay," she replied, this time with more confidence.

"So ... what do you want for dinner?" I had to change the subject before my heart burst wide open. The only thing worse than knowing your child is in pain, is to know that you are the cause of that pain.

When I arrived at her apartment I greeted her with a big smile and hugged her with all my might. I did a quick look up and down to make sure she was all right and then turned my attention to my grand-dog who was anxiously awaiting a hug from me, too. Remy jumped up on my legs, eyes wide, tail wagging with such enthusiasm it made me laugh.

"I see you, pretty girl. Did you miss me?" I rubbed her face between my hands then scooped her up in my arms. A flutter of doggy kisses went straight for my face and it was all I could do to keep them from landing anywhere close to my mouth. I put her down and went into the kitchen where my daughter was putting away groceries. Remy followed my every step.

"So, let's talk for a minute," I said. I wanted to

reassure her that I was fine … that *we* were going to be fine. And that despite the recent diagnosis, I was still mom and would continue to be mom in every way imaginable. I needed to remind her that we serve a mighty God and it is because of that faith I knew I was going to be all right. I told her how I had lost it in the car for a minute and then prayed. I explained to her that it was during that time of prayer that I had given the cancer over to God.

"I realized I've done everything I could do to prevent this from happening. From this point on it's out of my hands; all I can do now is trust God, so I'm not going to worry about it." I could tell by the look in her eyes she was frightened. "Do you have any questions, baby?"

"No," she said. "If you're not worried about it, then I'm not worried about it."

I would later learn that although she had put up a strong front that day, she *was* worried about it and had cried uncontrollably on several occasions thereafter.

My cell phone rang. It was Dr. Weston.

"Hi, Dr. Weston! How are you?"

"I'm fine, thank you. You sound in good spirits," she replied.

"I am! I spoke to Dr. Raine earlier, so I was just waiting for your call."

"Good. I know she told you about the diagnosis and I just wanted to reassure you that this is a highly treatable form of breast cancer. By catching it early the masses are small enough for you to have a lumpectomy, which you'll need to schedule as soon as possible. I want you to make an appointment with Dr. Flippiano; she's the best cancer surgeon in the area and I wouldn't want you to be seen by anyone else. Hear me now; even if you have to wait a couple of weeks to see her, wait; you have time." Her tone of voice put me at ease.

"That's good to hear because I have a trip planned to Honolulu Mother's Day week with my mom and daughter and I'm not going to miss it!" I replied matter-of-factly.

She laughed before responding. "Karrie, you amaze me. The cancer is not aggressive and you are young and strong. I don't see any reason for you to miss your trip."

"Young? Shoot, I'm almost fifty!" I said with a laugh.

The call ended with me knowing just enough information to quell my anxiety, but not enough to satisfy my need to know *why*. I relayed the information to my daughter and we put it behind us as best we could. From that moment on, my life and that of my daughter's would never be the same. The definition of what it meant to be us had just been rewritten … and there was nothing we could do about it except turn the page.

My Story: The Middle

Part 1

D r. Weston was right about Dr. Flippiano's popularity. Getting an appointment with her was like asking to see the President. I had exactly fourteen days before my appointment with her and twenty-one days before my trip to Honolulu, and I was anxious for both.

I hadn't told anyone about my diagnosis except my daughter. I hadn't fully come to terms with it because I still faithfully believed God for a miracle. In addition to that, I felt like a fraud. Why? For the past year and a half I had been promoting my first book, *Sweet Tea and Cornbread — Inspiring, Motivating and Empowering Black Women to Take Back Their Bodies and Live a Healthier Lifestyle*. How could I now announce to the world that I have cancer! How would I explain that everything I promoted in my book wasn't enough to prevent cancer from invading my body? I was embarrassed and I felt like a failure. In my book I make reference to a cousin who when asked why they didn't eat healthier said, "I could get hit by a car tomorrow, so I'm going to enjoy myself!" I thought about that cousin now; were they right? I had just devoted the last eight years of my life to creating the healthiest body I could, and had failed. At forty-eight years old I had managed to keep chronic disease and a life of maintenance drugs at bay, but had just been diagnosed with cancer. *How the heck does that happen?! Do you know how many hamburgers I've said no to and how many desserts I have passed up over the years trying to be healthy? It isn't fair!* The calories seemed insignificant now, and the exercise a waste of time. I went out that night full of self-pity and drove straight to McDonald's. I ordered the Big Mac combo, Sprite and two apple pies. That's right, *two!* As I placed the bag of food on the seat beside me, the familiar aroma of French fries filled the car and it was all I could do to keep from grabbing a handful, so I did. By the time I got home the fries were gone, but I ate the rest of my meal with a smile on my face, savoring every bite. Fifteen minutes, give or take a minute, after downing that dynamite, the explosion that took place in my stomach and the aftermath that ensued, left me and my colon regretful of my decision for the remainder of the evening.

Later that night I texted the news of my diagnosis to Pastor John and told him I had already anointed myself with oil, prayed and was feeling positive; all I needed from him was prayer. He responded back with shock and disbelief and asked if it was all right for him to share the news with the church. I told him no, that for now I wanted to keep it just between the two of us. He didn't press the issue and assured me he and his wife would keep me in their prayers. I know it probably sounds silly, keeping my condition private, but I wasn't ready for questions. I didn't want to see the looks on people's faces when they learned of the news, nor did I want their pity. I was preparing for battle and had enough to worry about without any negative vibes or criticism disturbing my camp.

I went to bible study that Wednesday night mentally exhausted and spiritually drained. I desperately needed to be recharged by the Word of God, and Pastor John didn't disappoint. The teaching that night took us on a trip that started in Romans and ended up in Genesis, Genesis 37, 39-50 to be exact, where we delved into the life of Joseph — The Pit, Potiphar's House and the Prison. The way Pastor John opened up the scripture and poured it into my heart set my spirit on fire! The Lord showed me that just like Joseph, I was going to have to go through some things before I could receive His promise, but if I kept my focus on Him and not the diagnosis, victory would be mine! Tears seeped into my eyes and I knew God was speaking directly to me. He had seen me praying on the floor in a puddle of tears. He had heard my thoughts of confusion, asking *why me!* He had felt my struggle to suppress my fears and had brought me here tonight to speak to my heart in a very unpretentious way, simply saying, "I'm here." Pastor John closed the class that evening by asking the church to pray and lay hands on me. He didn't say why and no one asked; they simply obeyed his request. I can still feel their love and the blanket of covering that came from their prayers. I wrapped it tight around my shoulders as I exited the church and walked to my car … I wore it all the way home.

I received a text from my cousin the next day, just chit chat, but it opened the door for me to reveal my secret to her. "*Can I call you?*" I typed the message and pushed send.

"*Sure!*" was her quick reply.

As soon as I heard her voice on the other end of my call a lump formed in my throat. I struggled to keep my composure; it didn't work. Thru the tears I sobbed the story of how I had just found out about the breast cancer.

"It's crazy, right? After all I've done to stay healthy, and now this happens!" I sobbed.

She shifted from younger cousin to the trained medical professional she is and began asking me questions. What type? Where was it located? What stage is it? I answered as best as I could, but even I didn't have all the answers. Her care and understanding helped ease the pain.

"I'm going to have to have surgery. I don't know when, but would you be able to come to the hospital just to be there with Korie? I'm sure she thinks she can handle everything by herself, but I don't want her to be alone."

"Of course! Just let me know when." Her response was typical of the caring person I've know her to be all her life.

"I haven't told my mom yet; do you think I should?" I questioned.

"What? You haven't told your mom? Why not?" she replied frantically.

"Because I don't want her to worry. I don't want her

to think she has to come out here and take care of me. I'm going to be fine," I said.

"I think Aunt Rose is strong enough to handle the news *and* I think she would be mad if you didn't tell her!" Her response was probably spot on when it came to my mother's reaction. We chatted a moment longer then said our goodbyes. I sat there reflecting on the conversation. Years before, her mother had lost her battle with cancer and now I was asking her to stand in the gap for me. Life — it twists and turns and makes absolutely no sense sometimes, but thank God for the angels he places in our lives at just the right moment.

I called my mom that evening, *No crying! No crying!* And I took a deep breath when she answered the call.

"Hello?" she said.

"Hi, Mom! Whatcha doin'?"

"Oh, I'm just packing. Trying to get ready for my trip to Denver. My group is going up to see a Rockies game," she replied.

"Oh, cool!" *That woman travels more than anyone I know!* 'Well … I was calling to tell you I just found out I have breast cancer, but don't worry, they caught it early. I'm meeting with a surgical oncologist in two weeks, so I'll know more then. Have fun on your trip! Call me when you get back!" *How was that for concise and upbeat?*

"What!" Her response confirmed I had failed. I proceeded with my brash attempt at calming her fears.

"I know! But there's no need to worry. I'm not! I've prayed about it and have given it to God, so the only thing I can do now is make my body as strong as I can. I've increased my workouts and I'm eating a more alkaline food diet so my body will be clean and strong by the time I have surgery. The only thing I need from you is prayer. Every-thing's going to be fine."

It really doesn't matter what she said next. What matters is that cancer had slithered its way into our lives yet again. This pernicious viper and the poisonous venom it carried came to test the resolve of our family when I was a child. Back then it attacked my father. He fought a valiant fight, but would go to rest with the Lord a few months later. As for now, I can only imagine the thoughts that ran through my mother's mind. Did she cry? Did she pray? Did she shout to the Lord? I did.

The two weeks until my appointment with Dr. Flippiano crept by at a snail's pace, which gave me plenty of time to work myself into a frenzy with all the stuff I had read about breast cancer on the internet. Instead of answering the questions I had, my research created more. I saw videos of people who had supposedly cured themselves with lemons and molasses, learned about a so-called superfruit from the rainforest that worked bonafied miracles, and everybody, it seemed, had a horror story to share about their experience with chemo or radiation therapy. On the day of my appointment I was armed with so much random infor-mation, I had become an expert in the obscure.

Dr. Flippiano's office was located in the Levine Cancer Institute. I remembered seeing the building on my last adventure to CMC-Main. I parked in the same deck as before and walked across the street to the front entrance of the building. As I crossed over the threshold into the lobby I was greeted by several young adults wearing navy blue shirts and khaki pants. One of the girls separated from the group and approached me with a big smile.

"Hello! Can I help you find something, ma'am?"

"I'm looking for Dr. Flippiano's office," I said, as I scanned the area. It was a beautiful facility. My decorator's eye appreciated the soothing, cool, aqua blue tones in the interior's color palette.

"Sure, no problem! Just take the elevator to the sixth floor," she replied, never dropping her smile.

"And then what?" I questioned, feeling like the most important part of the directions had been overlooked.

"As soon as you exit the elevator you'll see it," she answered confidently.

Okay. This could get interesting. "Thanks," I replied and made my way through the lobby to the elevators where I stopped behind a group of people waiting their turn. The elevator doors opened with a *ding* and I followed the rest of its passengers inside. I rode the five floors up alone with my thoughts. *You've got this! Be strong. Breathe! Why didn't I ask someone to come with me? Stupid, stupid!* My inner monologue was halted when the elevator doors opened onto the sixth floor. I stepped out into the hallway, looked right then left and saw the big sign on the wall just above a reception desk that read, Breast and Surgical Oncology Center. *Ha! She was right.* Down the hall to the left I would find the check-in and waiting area.

"There is a restroom and a beverage station just around the corner to the left with coffee, tea and water if you'd like anything," the receptionist announced after checking me in.

"I'm fine, thank you," I replied

"Do you have a parking ticket I can validate for you?" she asked.

"Ah, yes I do!" I reached into the black hole I call my purse and fished the ticket out. "Here you go."

She stamped the ticket and handed it back to me. "Just have a seat and I'll bring your paperwork over to you."

"Thank you," I said and took a seat near the windows.

The waiting area was not overly crowded; there were just a handful of men and women waiting for their various appointments. I noticed that some of them wore wigs, some wore scarves or hats and some of them, like me, had full heads of hair. *I wonder if the fact that I still have my hair classifies me as a freshman. Would I eventually graduate to wearing a scarf or hat?* Before I could worry myself any further a nurse walked thru the door and announced my name. "Karrie Marchbanks?" I grabbed my purse and the paperwork they had given me and followed her back to the examination room.

After disrobing from the waist up and changing into the hospital gown, I settled into a chair and prepared for a long wait, which actually only turned out to be maybe a minute or two.

"Ms. Marchbanks? Hi, my name is Nicole. How are you?"

"I'm fine, considering."

"I know. Well, I'm going to take your vitals and ask you a few questions, okay?" She went through the standard routine — height, weight, blood pressure, temperature, etc. Then she asked me what medications I was taking. I told her none. She asked again and I told her none … again.

"I'm sorry, I don't get that response very often; I'm

used to people pulling out a list of meds as long as their arm. I just wanted to make sure," she replied with a laugh.

I laughed with her and said, "No problem; I get that a lot, too." *I would be in perfect health if I didn't have breast cancer.*

There would be one more nurse for me to see before Dr. Flippiano arrived. She told me she was my Patient Coordinator and handed me a large three ring binder full of information about my diagnosis, treatment options and the institute itself. She told me that my care would include genetic testing to rule out any future risk for me or my family, and nutritional support with a registered dietician to discuss which foods to avoid as well as those foods that will increase my energy and support my immune system. She showed me a calendar with dates and times of support groups, yoga classes and massage therapy slots, if I felt so inclined. It was all a bit overwhelming, but at the same time incredible that they had created a treatment plan that considered the whole person, as well as their family, and not just the disease.

By the time Dr. Flippiano arrived my head was swimming. She entered the room with a smile and reached out to shake my hand. She was about average height, her blond hair streaked with gray, but it didn't make her look old; instead, it suited her. She wore large diamond studs in her ears, which I thought was a bit cocky of her, and I liked it! *Not only could she kick your butt in the operating room; she looked good doing it!* She stood for a moment while we greeted each other then sat down at a desk with two computer monitors. I sat beside her. She went into my patient history and pulled up the results of my mammogram. Once again I came face-to-face with the four white spots, and honestly, I was getting pretty tired of seeing them. Dr. Flippiano explained everything about my cancer in such detail I felt like I was in medical school. She used the computer in front of her to draw out the surgical procedure, and explained with words I could actually comprehend how having a lumpectomy would affect my body immediately after surgery and in the future. She told me that my specific type of cancer wouldn't require chemotherapy; instead, I would undergo radiation treatments as determined by yet another specialist — a doctor of radiation oncology. She wrapped up the dissertation by saying, "So, that's it. You're lucky it was caught early and because you're young and in good health, I don't foresee any complications. You'll come through this with no problems. Do you have any questions for me? Is there anything you would like me to go over again?"

"I only have one question," I said. "How did this happen? I've done everything I know of to take care of myself and yet I'm sitting here having this conversation with you. I need to know why."

"Karrie," she said, "If I knew that, I would be out of a job. There are the obvious factors like genetics or smoking, but there are also the unknown factors that we're still researching today. As far as I can tell from your medical history, genetics doesn't play a role, but you'll have an opportunity to discuss that further with the counselor. You were born a woman and that alone puts you at risk."

Trying to absorb all the information I received that day was next to impossible. It was all so surreal! I half expected Ashton Kutcher to burst through the door, camera crew in tow, and tell me I had just been punked! I told her about my trip to Honolulu and how I wanted to postpone the surgery until I got back.

"I don't have a problem waiting a couple more

weeks, but I wouldn't put it off any longer than that," she said. So we scheduled the pre-op appointment for the day after my return.

My mind and body felt numb as I left the building and walked back to my car. The heat from the sun felt good against my cool skin. I sat in my car for a moment reflecting on what Dr. Flippiano had just told me. *She said I was lucky.* I guess if you look at it from a medical perspective I was, indeed, lucky. The number of people who continue to die from treatable cancers in America is a tragedy and for African American women the numbers are even worse. But I knew that luck had nothing to do with the early detection of my breast cancer and *everything* to do with God! He was the one who whispered into my ear two months after I had failed to schedule my annual mammogram and told me to make the appointment. And He was the one who cleared the calendar that day at four o'clock to open a slot for me. If it wasn't for the Holy Spirit speaking to me that day, I might not even be here! But He did, and I listened and I thank Him every day for loving me so much He took time out of His very busy schedule to consider me.

I drove home that day determined not to focus on the surgery, but on the upcoming trip. This Mother's Day was going to be extra special; I was sure of that!

My Story: The Middle

Part 2

Honolulu was amazing! Our hotel was a gorgeous property on the beautiful Waikiki Beachwalk just about a block from the white sands of beautiful Waikiki beach. From our balconies we had a magnificent view of the ocean and Diamond Head in the distance, and front row seats to the bustling night life on the streets of the Beachwalk below. We ate, we shopped, we toured, and we laughed, simply enjoying each other's company. We made memories that we'll laugh about and cherish forever. But the significance of the trip wasn't lost in all the revelry; God had strengthened the bond between the generations and we will forever be grateful for every opportunity we have together while on this earth.

The flight back to the mainland took thirteen hours. My daughter and I landed at Charlotte Douglas Airport with only an hour left before my pre-op appointment with Dr. Flippiano. We hurried home; I showered, changed and jumped back in the car, determined not to be late. *I could have sworn I had made the appointment for the day after we got back!* I arrived at the hospital glowing on the outside from my new Hawaiian tan and renewed on the inside from witnessing God's majesty in nature up close and personal. The receptionist noticed right away.

"Hi, Ms. Marchbanks! You look like you got a little sun!" she said with a smile.

"No, I got a lot of sun! I just got back from a trip to Honolulu an hour ago," I replied with a laugh.

"And you didn't take me with you? Must be nice," she said. "Just have a seat and they'll call you back shortly." The meeting with Dr. Flippiano was for informational purposes only. She told me what to expect the day of the surgery and to make sure I had someone to drive me home after the procedure.

"Because of the side effects from the anesthesia, you'll need someone to stay with you for at least twenty-four hours; forty-eight would be even better; you can't be too careful. And no heavy lifting for a couple of days; just take it easy." The tone in her voice sounded as if she knew my independent streak all too well. She explained the necessity of monitoring my post surgery breast with follow up exams and more frequent mammograms, and then we scheduled the surgery for Thursday of the following week. *Wow! So soon?* The appointment lasted only a few minutes and then I was back in my car, left alone with my fear. *I don't want to do this! I don't want to be this person! I want my normal, healthy body back!*

Please, Lord! Just then, a song came on the radio; it was unfamiliar to me, but the words were like salve to my broken spirit:

> *Even though I can't see*
> *and I can't feel your touch*
> *I will trust you, Lord*
> *how I love you so much*
> *though my nights may seem long*
> *and I feel so alone*
> *Lord, my trust is in you*
> *I surrender to you.*

I cried for a moment, my mind feverishly trying to process everything I had just been told. I had known cancer to be a death sentence, or at the very least a very traumatic and devastating course of treatment to have to go through. So to now become one of the thousands to receive this diagnosis frightened me. I prayed and asked God to forgive me for being so weak. I was trying so hard to stay positive, but with every new procedure my flesh gave way to fear.

I drove slowly back to the house, trying to regain my composure, and by the time I arrived I was ready to be Mom again and spend the next couple of hours with my daughter before she made her way back to Savannah. My mother called later that evening to let me know she had arrived home safely and then asked about my appointment. I explained what Dr. Flippiano said and assured her there was no need for her to unpack, re-pack and catch a flight out to Charlotte the very next week … that with my daughter coming back and my cousin standing watch, I was in good hands.

The week leading up to the surgery flew by! Between work, church, the gym, grocery shopping and trying to clean every inch of the house and car before I went under the knife, I was tired. Some people would call it obsessive; I call it prepared. I wanted to make sure that in case it took longer to recuperate than expected, I wouldn't have to worry about anything but getting better. Plus, it gave my mind something to focus on instead of dwelling on the what ifs. The fear of being under anesthesia, knocked out and not in control was freaking me out. The anxiety of it all led me to call my cousin and tell her where to find my Will and the insurance papers in the event that something went wrong.

"Don't tell me!" she said. "Tell Korie! I don't want to hear that. Besides, you're gonna be fine."

The night before my surgery I went to Bible study and before we could even get started good Pastor John asked everyone to pray and lay hands on me. In his passion and faith in the Word of God, his prayer revealed the secret I had kept for two months to the rest of the congregation — I had breast cancer. Apprehension set in as I opened my eyes and looked around, but instead of judgment I saw concern. Instead of mockery I received compassion. I saw my church. I saw love. That night, I shared what I had been going through with a couple of my spiritual sisters and for the first time since the diagnosis, felt a sense of relief because of the burden their love had lifted from my shoulders. More than I would ever admit to, I so desperately needed their encouragement and support during this test of faith.

The teaching that night took us to Matthew 14:21-34. Pastor John brought the story to life in such a way that he might as well have been talking about me, for just as the disciples were shaken by the storm and Peter, whose faith would be tested, Jesus was asking me to step out of the boat and put my trust in Him against the storm which swirled around me now. He was standing there, holding out His hand. Would I hold fast to His gaze or be distracted by the winds and fall?

I spent the rest of the evening with my daughter, her boyfriend, who had made the trip with her, and my grand-dog. We talked and laughed and played games with Remy until she called it quits and retired to her crate. I wanted to enjoy my family as long as I could, but I knew they were tired from the long drive, so I said goodnight and headed upstairs to bed. Tomorrow was the big day, and although I'm sure God would have understood if I focused tonight's prayers on me and my situation, I thought about Peter and chose not to be distracted by the winds and prayed a prayer of thanks, instead. *Thank you, Lord, for all the blessings you have given me and those I have yet to see. Thank you, Lord, for guiding me through this very difficult process with your mighty hand. You are my Lord and Savior, my provider, my protector, my strength and my love. Without you I am nothing! Thank you for the angel you sent to guide my daughter safely home today and Lord, please comfort my family tomorrow; give them peace of mind and please watch over my daughter; she needs you. In Jesus' name I pray, Amen.*

The day of the surgery I was a bundle of nerves. I woke up with peace about the procedure, but full of questions just the same, and I was tired of them leaving their footprints of doubt across my brain for me to have to clean up later. I was ready to get past this phase and on to the next one. The emotional ups and downs had taken their toll.

Would it hurt, would I be in pain? What if I'm one of those people who are only asleep and not completely knocked out and I feel everything? What if ...What if! I had been standing in my closet staring straight ahead at all the clothes for I don't know how long and yet saw nothing. Eventually, the fog lifted and I settled on a pair of black capris with a drawstring, a white button up shirt and a pair of red, beaded flip flops with a cork bottom. I laughed at the thought of my daughter trying to help dress me in the event I couldn't manage it on my own and figured I would try to make it as easy as possible for her.

There was an uneasy quiet in the house that morning. And I secretly wished my daughter hadn't come. I didn't know how I was going to feel after surgery and I didn't want her to have to see me struggling and in pain. I thought back to when I was a child and to seeing my father frail and helpless as he lay in the hospital bed dying of cancer. I didn't want her to feel that pain, to see me in a state of helplessness. *I'm the mom; I'm supposed to take care of her, not the other way around.* So, I did what any mother would do; I carried the burden. I tried to make jokes and talked about the weather, anything to lighten the mood, anything to keep her happy, but my attempts fell flat. The pink elephant in the room had parked itself right in front of our happiness, and I think I just saw it pick up a magazine.

Traffic was a nightmare! Several detours and one stop at Starbucks later, we finally arrived at the outpatient surgery center of CMC-Main. I was a pro now at navigating through the hospital and, much to my daughter's chagrin, made reference to various points of interest along our way through the building.

"See, it has its own pharmacy! And on the fifth floor there's a Chick-fil-A! And, oh, that's the lady I told you about with the Jamaican accent." My daughter and her boyfriend obliged my nerves with a smile on their faces and the occasional nod of the head until we arrived in front of the reception desk and reality set in. Check-in went rather quickly. They banded my wrist with an identification bracelet and then gestured to the waiting area where we all took seats near a television to wait for the nurse. The small talk continued until I noticed my cousin approaching from the distance. I stood up to greet her with a hug.

"Hi! Thank you so much for coming!" I felt better already. She made her rounds; passing out hugs to everyone then took a seat beside me.

"So, how long have you been waiting?" she asked.

"Not long. I'm anxious to get this over with, though." And just as the words left my mouth, Dr. Flippiano came through a set of double doors and walked over to where we were sitting.

"Hi, Karrie. I just wanted to come out and let you know we're just about ready for you. Is this your family?"

"Hi! Yes. Dr. Flippiano, this is my cousin, Cindy, my daughter, Korie and her boyfriend, Travis," I replied proudly.

"You two look like sisters!" she said, pointing at my daughter. "Well, it was so nice to meet you all. It shouldn't be much longer. I'll see you in the back." And with that, she disappeared behind the same doors she had entered.

A few minutes later a nurse appeared and called my name. I rose from my seat, turned and gave my daughter a hug.

"See you in a little bit, baby. I love you!" I said, trying my best not to become emotional.

"Oh, she'll see you again," the nurse said. "I'll come back to get everyone after we prep you."

"Oh, wow; I had no idea! Great, so I *will* see you in a little bit." I laughed, and turned to follow the nurse through the doors. *Here we go, no turning back now.*

The behind-the-scenes action in an outpatient surgery center can best be described as orchestrated pandemonium. I had never seen anything like it except on TV. Doctors, nurses, and patients ... oh my! People were everywhere and I was about to become part of the bedlam. I was led to a room of sorts, more like a cubby with a curtain, and was told to have a seat and wait for the nurse. I sat there watching the commotion while the anxiety rose in my chest. The nurse entered the room and I didn't even see her.

"Hi. Ms. Marchbanks? I'm Anna. I'm going to ask you a few questions and then I'm going to give you a gorgeous outfit, complete with hat and slippers to wear to surgery. Okay?" she said with a laugh.

"Okaaay." I replied and smiled.

I admired her for her light heartedness and sense of humor. She had probably witnessed some pretty traumatic things over the years, but was able to keep it all in perspective. She sat down on a stool in front of a computer and began the litany of questions. When she came to the part about what kind of medications I was taking, I once again had to explain twice.

"You're not taking *any* medication?" she questioned.

"No. Only my supplements," I replied.

She looked back to the computer and clicked through the pages in an attempt to confirm I was mistaken, but when she couldn't find any evidence to the contrary, shook her head and said, "Wow, I don't see that very often, especially in adults. What are you doing here?" She joked.

"Exactly!" I replied, and she reached over, grabbed a

hospital gown, what looked like a shower cap and a pair of non-slip socks out of a cabinet and handed them to me. She turned and pointed to a stick figure cartoon drawing hanging on the wall adjacent to where I was sitting, of a man wearing the same items of clothing she had just given to me.

"When you get everything on you should look like this! Except of course you'll still be a lady." She laughed. She gave me a mesh bag in which to put my personal affects and left the room, closing the curtain behind her. *Here we go. You can do this. Everything's going to be alright,* I thought as my heart raced faster.

A few minutes later another nurse arrived to take me back to have my breast mapped for surgery. During the lumpectomy Dr. Raine had implanted two surgical clips marking the spot of the cancer. They would now locate those clips using a type of x-ray machine and then draw an X on my skin to mark the surgical site. The procedure took a few minutes and I was surprised to see Dr. Flippiano, who stopped by to make sure everything was correct. She looked very different in the blue surgical scrubs she now wore — powerful and very official and I was glad she would be performing my surgery. Afterwards, I was taken back to my cubby to wait for the anesthesiologist.

The nurse who performed the intake came back to insert a central line into my hand and shortly after that the anesthesiologist arrived and introduced himself. He explained what his role was and checked to see if I was on any medication.

"Why do *you* need to know if I'm taking medication?" I asked.

"Because if you are, I might need to adjust the amount or type of anesthesia I give you. For example, if you are taking medication for, let's say, high blood pressure, I would know to monitor your blood pressure very closely and watch for any side effects from the anesthesia."

The nurse chimed in. "She's not on any meds, doctor." And then she turned and spoke to me. "You don't have to worry about a thing. You're in good health and you don't have any chronic diseases; you make our jobs easy!"

After the doctor left, the nurse asked me if I would like for her to bring my family back. I told her, "Yes," and moments later she returned with my daughter and cousin.

"Where's Travis?" I asked my daughter, surprised at his absence.

"He went to take a call," she replied.

"What? I wanted him to pray before they knock me out!" Travis is an elder and I was hoping to have the extra covering from his prayers.

"We can wait for you to go get him," the nurse said to my daughter.

"No, it's okay. I'm ready," I said, then gave my daughter and cousin a hug before telling them once again that I loved them as they exited the room.

A gurney arrived and the nurse helped me maneuver myself onto it before attaching a saline bag to the line in my hand. She gave me a shot of something to help me relax and wheeled me out of the cubby and down the hall toward the operating room. I lay there, nervously chatting away, making random conversation about anything and everything, wondering anxiously when that shot was going to kick in. The nurse leaned over and smiled at me and said, "Relax; let the medicine do its job." Reluctantly, I stopped talking, closed my eyes and started to pray. *Our Father who art in hea…*

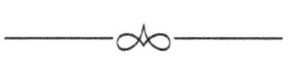

"Karrie … Ms. Marchbanks…" A voice called out from the distance. My eyes struggled to open then quickly closed under the weight of the anesthesia.

"Ms. Marchbanks…" There it was again, beckoning me from beyond. I pried my eyes open and slowly looked around. The people laying in beds against the wall to my right suggested I was in the post-op ward and not in heaven; the nurse standing at the foot of my bed asking me annoying questions confirmed it. I ignored her intrusive quest for information and focused in on the clock on the wall behind her. *Had it really been six hours since I arrived?* I looked to the nurse, who was still asking questions, then down to my chest. I had expected to see bandages, but instead saw a funny looking white bra with cups way bigger than I would ever need. *When did they put this on me?* I pulled it back, away from my chest and saw gauze bandages taped to my skin.

"The surgery went fine; you did very well. We're going to keep you in post-op for awhile until you come out of the anesthesia, then I'll move you to a recovery room. How do you feel?"

I tried to open my mouth to speak and realized my lips were swollen and my throat was in a lot of pain. *Did they take my tonsils out, too?* With as little effort as possible I struggled to explain this to the nurse. She nodded in agreement, then walked away and returned with an ice pack.

"Here you go. Hold this to your mouth; it will help reduce the swelling," she instructed.

My body felt heavy and I drifted in and out of sleep for several more minutes before the nurse decided it was okay for me to be moved. She helped me out of the bed and into a wheelchair, and then pushed me out of the room past the other post-opees and down a short hallway to a cubby with a recliner, a chair and a bench. I made the transition from the wheelchair to the recliner unassisted and she covered me with a warm blanket. As soon as she left, the recovery nurse came in and checked the saline drip. She told me she was going to increase the fluids to help speed the recovery process.

"Also, let me know if you start to get nauseous because I can add something to the drip to make it stop. Okay?"

I wasn't ready to try talking again, so I nodded my head in agreement and closed my eyes, my body immediately overcome with sleep.

The sound of familiar voices interrupted a very peaceful slumber and I opened my eyes just in time to see my daughter and cousin enter the small room. I smiled at the sight of them.

"Hi, Lovie! I'm still alive." My voice sounded raspy as I croaked out the words. I tried swallowing, but to no avail since my mouth was as dry as burnt toast. "My throat is killing me and look at my lips! Aren't they huge?"

"They're not that big," she said, trying her best to sound positive. I could see the concern for my wellbeing in her eyes, and I was glad my cousin had been there for support. Her eyes traveled from my face to the line in my hand and up to the saline bag.

The nurse chimed in, "It's probably from the tube they used to intubate you; it will go away. In the meantime, I need to get you to eat something before you can be released; do you think you're ready to try?"

"I'll try, but I won't like it," I said, while rubbing my throat. She came back with a pack of saltine crackers and half a cup of warm Coke — probably the two worst things you can give a person with dry mouth and a sore throat, but I did my best to get as much down as I could.

Seeing that I was all right, and in capable hands with my daughter sitting by my side, my cousin said her goodbyes and told me she would call later to check on me. The nurse came in and attached a second bag of saline to the line, which minutes later proved to be just enough water to send my bladder over the edge and open the flood gates. I had to pee, like now! I asked my daughter to call for the nurse, and as soon as she helped me to my feet a wave of nausea hit me with such force it almost brought me to my knees. I thought I was going to lose it right there, but the nurse helped steady my walk and I was able to make it to the bathroom and back to the chair without incident.

"Let me go get the anti-nausea medicine; it'll make you feel better and help ease your symptoms. I'll be right back."

When she returned she added the liquid to the saline bag and told me I should feel better momentarily. She was right. I closed my eyes as the medicine started to take effect, and drifted in and out of sleep for several more minutes until I was feeling much better. Shortly thereafter, they decided it was okay for me to get dressed and my daughter helped me on with my clothes.

"You made the right decision when you put this outfit together," she said as she buttoned up my shirt and slid the flip flops onto my feet.

Dr. Flippiano stopped by to tell me the initial lab tests revealed that she was successful in removing all the cancer, but that she would call me later with more information and to check up on me.

"Thank you, Jesus! And thank you, Dr. Flippiano, for everything," I said.

"You're so very welcome. I want to see you in a couple of weeks for a follow up, so look for a call from scheduling," she said before leaving the room.

That was the best news I had received all day and I was ready to get out of there and go home. Taking the doctor's departure as my cue to leave, I rose from my chair and stood up.

"And where do you think you're going?" the nurse asked, as if I were a child who was trying to leave the table before finishing their vegetables. Apparently it's protocol to ride in a wheelchair after surgery, so I returned to my seat like a good little girl and waited for her to bring my transportation.

"I'll go get the car and bring it around," my daughter said, and she hurriedly left the room.

The nurse arrived moments later with my silver chariot and insisted on helping me transfer to its waiting seat. The room spun as a wave of nausea hit me once again, but I wasn't about to let on and miss my opportunity to go home.

"Feet on the paddles," she instructed, and we were off, snaking our way through the ward until we reached the exit door. My daughter pulled up to the curb just as the doors parted and the nurse wheeled me outside.

The sun was bright to my sleepy eyes, but its warmth felt good on my face. I took a deep breath of the warm air to help clear the cobwebs from my head, then rose from my seat and stepped into the waiting car. I turned and waved to the nurse as we pulled away from the curb.

"Let's pick up Chinese on the way home; I'm starving!" I said to my daughter.

"How about I take you home and then *we'll* go get Chinese food," she said, pointing her thumb toward the back seat at Travis. I laughed to myself. My baby had just made it known that *she* was head of the house now, so I sat back in the seat, closed my eyes and let her love take control.

I slept for about two hours, and so soundly I didn't know whether they had made it back or not so I grabbed my phone off the nightstand and texted her to see where she was. As I watched the phone, waiting for her response, the motion of the bedroom door swinging open almost scared me to death until I saw her standing there with a smile on her face. She walked over to the bed and gingerly sat down beside me.

"How do you feel?" The look of concern on her face told me she was expecting the worst.

I was still a little groggy from the anesthesia and it was still very hard for me talk, but I gave it a try. "Actually, I feel good. The only thing that hurts is my throat, but I'm so hungry I don't even care. Would you bring me something to eat and some water, please? My mouth is so dry."

"Are you sure you're ready to eat? How does your stomach feel?" she asked cautiously.

"Baby, I haven't eaten since yesterday! Yes, I'm ready."

Reluctantly, she left the room then returned with a plate of saltine crackers and a mini can of ginger ale.

"What happened to the Chinese food? I thought you were going to go get food when you dropped me off?"

"We did. Try eating this first and see how you do." The power had gone to her head! She was taking this nurse thing a little too far, but I was in no position to argue, so I choked down my six crackers and sipped my ginger ale without further protest.

"Now can I have some real food, please?" I asked, trying to sound as contrite as I possibly could to avoid further punishment. This time she returned with a plate — a rather small plate of sesame chicken, fried rice and a glass of water. My stomach growled at the smell of the food. I took a bite of the chicken and chewed it slowly. It was so good, but I had no idea how I was going to swallow it when the time came. The pain the food caused as it squeezed down my throat felt like I had just swallowed a mouth full of rocks and I was seriously afraid I had just done severe damage. I took a drink of water to help lubricate the tight passage and help ease the friction, but it didn't work. I would have called it quits right then and there if I weren't so stubborn ... I mean hungry.

Nurse Korie came back to take my dishes and to ask if I needed any pain pills.

"No, I'm not in any pain at all. But leave the bottle and a glass of water on the nightstand just in case I need it later." The fogginess in my head and the heaviness in my body brought sleep once again and when I closed my eyes for what would be the last time that evening, I slept peacefully, oblivious to the events that had started the day.

I woke the next day feeling so much better; I was ready to get out of bed and do something, anything! It was time for me to regain my position at the head of the family and I could think of no better way to do that than with the homemade pancakes my daughter loved the most, so I threw on a pair of sweat pants and a t-shirt and went downstairs. She looked surprised to see me when I appeared around the corner and Remy ran over to greet me, bouncing with excitement.

"What are you doing out of bed? How do you feel?" she asked.

"Actually, I feel pretty good. A little tired, but still no pain, so that's a good thing."

"Did you take any medicine? How's your throat?"

"My throat still hurts, but I haven't felt the need to take any medicine. I'm going to fix pancakes; do you want some?" As if I didn't already know the answer.

She protested mildly, just for show, then relinquished her authority and handed over the keys to the kingdom.

The burst of energy that made me think I was Superwoman early that morning was short lived, and although I still wasn't experiencing any pain, the cooking and conversation had worn me out; it was time to take a nap. I didn't want to leave my family, so I lay down on the couch while they watched TV. It was Saturday and my daughter had to go back to Savannah in time for work the next day, but she doted on me until the last minute. She whizzed around the house making sure everything was clean and taken care of before they left. I lay there watching her, and for the first time in twenty-four years my eyes didn't see a little girl anymore. They saw the capable and caring grown woman she had become and I thought to myself, *I'm so glad God chose me to be her mother.*

My Story: The Beginning

Part 1

Sunday morning arrived and I woke up anxious to go to church. My throat was almost back to normal and I still hadn't experienced any real pain, just soreness; it felt like I had been punched in the chest rather than recovering from surgery. I hadn't come out of the hospital bra since they put it on me and now, standing in front of the bathroom mirror, I was nervous to see what lied beneath it as I opened the front clasp and let it slide down over my arms. Dr. Flippiano had told me the stitches would dissolve over time and I could see them now as I slowly pulled back the white gauze pads. The scar wasn't as big as I had imagined, only about an inch and a half in length, but it was very bruised and swollen. I laughed when I looked at myself in the mirror and saw the big black *X* and the word, *Yes*, still inscribed on my breast. *That would make one hilarious tattoo!* I stood there for a moment gazing at the new me. Sure, the scar would be a constant reminder of the cancer that had invaded my breast, but unlike so many other women who have fought their own battles with cancer, I still had a breast. I decided right then and there that when I looked at my scar I would not see pain and fear. No, my scar was a reminder of God's mercy and love, a testament to my faith and survival a badge of courage, and I would wear it proudly.

After a relaxing hot shower, I threw on a pink and purple print sundress and grabbed a white cardigan to keep me warm in the cool air conditioned church. I took the ice pack out of the freezer just before I left and tucked it inside my bra. The doctor hadn't told me to continue treating the area, but I had come to the conclusion that the ice pack was responsible for keeping the pain to a minimum, so I continued to use it, at least for one more day.

It felt good to be out of the house and to feel the breeze blowing through the open windows as I drove down the highway. Like any other Sunday, I used the forty-five minute drive to conduct my own praise and worship service, and by the time I turned into the parking lot of the church my spirit was re-energized and I was feeling good!

The harmonious sound of the praise team greeted me as I entered the church and took a seat near the back; the presence of God was palpable. Moments later Pastor John took his place behind the podium and started to pray. When he opened his eyes and looked out into the crowd he saw me standing there and smiled.

"Some of you don't know this because she didn't want me to say anything, but if you want to know how good God is, turn around and look at Sister Karrie. This woman of God had surgery to remove breast cancer on Thursday and is standing here in church today, three days later! You can't tell me God isn't good!"

The congregation erupted in praise, clapping and shouting. I felt the rush of the Holy Spirit enter my body and started to weep. I received so many hugs that day, and a few admonishments for being out so soon after surgery, but I counted it all joy because I was there, alive and was ready to give God all the glory and praise He deserved.

I went back to work on Monday and back to see Dr. Flippiano on Thursday, one week after the surgery. The stitches hadn't completely come out, but I was more worried about a noticeable dent that had formed presumably where she had removed the cancer.

"That's completely normal," she said. "As you continue to heal the area will fill in, the scar will improve and the swelling will go away. I see no signs of infection, so I'd say you're making good progress."

"So when can I go back to the gym?" I had moved past the breast exam and wanted to talk about more important things.

Dr. Flippiano raised her eyebrows and said, "You realize you're only a week out from surgery, right? You've got to be careful right now; your body is still healing. I wouldn't want you to pick up an infection and reverse all the progress you've made. But, with that said, I know how determined you are and if you promise you won't lift any weights, I would agree to some light exercise, and I mean light!"

"I promise! Thank you, Dr. Flippiano! You don't know how anxious I am to get back to my routine," I said with a smile. She told me she wanted to see me again in two weeks and to expect a call from scheduling to book the appointment with the radiation oncologist.

"They usually don't start radiation treatments until three weeks out to give your body time to recover, but they'll want to meet with you now to discuss treatment options," she explained.

I left the office with a spirit of thankfulness, smiling and saying hello to everyone who walked by. I had no clue how long the radiation treatments would take or how they would affect my body, but right now, in this moment, I was on top of the world!

Over the next few weeks my body continued to heal from the surgery. Matter of fact, if it were not for the scar, there would have been no physical evidence of the life changing events that had taken place just weeks before. From the mammogram to the diagnosis, to the biopsy and the surgery, there had been cancer in my body and now it was gone. I felt so good I began to question why the doctors were so eager for me to undergo radiation. *If the cancer is gone, why do I have to subject my body to the risks of radiation?* I was frightened by the thought of it and was seriously considering not going through with it at all.

As typical of my analytical personality, I needed to know more about this procedure, so I turned to the internet to research the subject and found website after website on the topic, plus more images of the side effects than my eyes wanted to see. There were pictures of people whose skin had become blackened or blistered after weeks of radiation treatments, and, as if that weren't enough, they shared their stories about the pain they endured and the ineffectiveness of the topical creams that were specifically designed to soothe the damaged skin. *Lord, I don't want to do this. I can't do this! How am I supposed to go to treatment everyday and work, too? It's too much.* I was scared and had come to the conclusion that radiation was not going to be part of my treatment plan, but there was that little nagging inside, that little seed of doubt that maybe my decision was wrong, so I looked to my friends and family for support. I knew that with them on my side I could walk into that doctor's office and tell him I was not having radiation and proclaim my faith in the healing power of God with confidence. At least that was my plan. You know the old saying, *"Don't ask if you really don't want to know the answer."* Well, the more I tried to convince them I shouldn't do it, the more reasons they came up with as to why I should, and by the end of the week I was more confused than ever. Then I realized that the only person I hadn't asked for guidance was Jesus. So I prayed. *Dear Lord, I'm afraid and I need your help. Give me a spirit of discernment, Lord, to help me figure out what to do. Fill me with your Holy Spirit and speak to me, Lord. Speak to my ears so that I can hear you, speak to my heart so that I can feel you, and give me eyes to see, Lord, so I will know that it is you! You are my Lord and Savior; I can't do this without you. Speak to me, Lord; speak to my heart. I bless your Holy name! In Jesus Christ I pray, Amen!*

The day of my appointment with the radiation oncologist I still wasn't sure what to do, but tried not to worry about it. God always comes in His perfect timing. I backed the car out of the driveway and heard the sound of my audio bible begin to play. The music began and the narrator's booming voice said, "The book of Psalms continued." Psalms chapter fifty-six began to play and as I listened to the words I knew my prayers had been answered. The verse concluded with the following scripture.

"I praise God for what he has promised;
yes, I praise the LORD for what he has promised."

"I trust in God, so why should I be afraid?
What can mere mortals do to me?"

"I will fulfill my vows to you, O God,
and will offer a sacrifice of thanks for your help."

"For you have rescued me from death;
you have kept my feet from slipping.
So now I can walk in your presence, O God,
in your life-giving light."

That was it! I had my answer. Truly, God had saved me from death, so why wouldn't He protect me from this, too? He promised me a victory, so there was nothing to fear.

"Thank you, Jesus!" I shouted out loud and began to praise Him and ask His forgiveness for the doubts that had captured my trust. I wiped the tears from my eyes as I pulled into the hospital's parking lot and then sat there for a minute and continued to listen to the bible's message before exiting the car. Doubt had been replaced with confidence and trust and I was ready to proceed with the next leg of this journey — the radiation treatments.

Dr. Bobian's office was located in the Pineville Radiation Therapy Center on the first floor of the CMC-Medical Plaza. I met with him for about twenty minutes as we discussed everything from my cancer, the surgery and the type of radiation therapy that was recommended for women with my diagnosis. He went over the treatment plan thoroughly and even humored my attempt at bargaining down the number of weeks of therapy from seven to five. He wasn't convinced, so for six weeks I would have a standing appointment at the center for treatments, Monday through Friday, but on the seventh week he would administer a more intense, localized boost of radiation for three days instead of five. When it was all said and done I would have received a total of thirty-three radiation treatments.

That same day in preparation for the upcoming treatments, they mapped my upper torso, using a type of 3-D MRI machine and I received my first *tattoos*. The radiation therapist made six permanent ink dots around my breast using the coordinates from the MRI to map the radiation field. The ink burned a little as it entered my skin through the thin needle, but the discomfort lasted only a few seconds. These markings would act as points of origin for each treatment going forward. Then she took a pink highlighter and drew a line around to each dot, connecting them as she went along. When she had finished I could clearly see the area to be treated, and it was comforting to know it wasn't as big as I had imagined. I also received a body mold of the position of my arms as they lay resting outstretched above my head. This mold was another safeguard used to ensure the accuracy of every treatment. What followed next was a tour of the facility, the women's changing room and instructions on how to use the computer to check-in. A print out of a calendar showing my appointment times was the last handout I would be given before I left the facility. I went home that afternoon with a complete understanding of what

I had just committed to, but I could not in a million years have known the magnitude of how my decision would transform not only my body, but my entire world.

My Story: The Beginning

Part 2

There were ten days left until the treatments began and massive doses of radiation entered my breast with one goal, complete annihilation, so I went on the offensive, determined to make the rest of my body as strong as possible. In addition to my workouts, supplements and twice daily vegetable smoothies, Dr. Bobian had prescribed a topical skin cream designed to hydrate the skin and minimize the damage caused by the radiation. His instructions were to apply it twice a day once the treatments began, but I decided to start using it immediately. My theory was this: if the purpose of the cream was to draw moisture to the damaged tissues, why not hydrate the area as much as possible before treatments began to help delay the side effects? Seemed logical to me, but only time would tell if my theory was sound, so I began applying the cream three times a day until my first treatment.

July sixteenth, just ten days after my forty-ninth birthday, I arrived at the office in good spirits. Sure, I was nervous, but I was trying really hard not to dwell on it. *Only thirty-three treatments. I can do this, right?* The receptionist greeted me as I approached the desk.

"Hi, Ms. Marchbanks. There's no need to check in with us; from now on just walk through to the changing room and check-in on the computer in the back."

"Oh, okay. Thanks," I replied and walked around to the door leading to women's changing room. The room had a small waiting area with a TV, a bathroom and two changing stalls enclosed with curtains. Stall number two was already occupied, so I entered the other stall and pulled the curtain closed. There were four locked cabinets in the little room and I claimed number two as my locker of choice for the duration. There was a cabinet filled with hospital gowns up above to the left, so I grabbed one, undressed from the waist up and slid the gown up over my arms, this time opening to the back. With my valuables securely locked away, I stepped out of the room and walked around to the computer to sign myself in. The number of names that appeared on the screen took me by surprise. The calendar was filled from morning till evening with the names of men and women who had appointments for treatment. I found my name on the second page and clicked the box.

No sooner had I taken a seat, the therapist walked through the door and called my name. "Ms. Marchbanks? We're ready for you."

My heart beat faster. "Wow! That was quick," I said with a nervous laugh. *I didn't even have time to pray.* I followed her out of the room and as I started to go left, she went right.

"Oh, no, Ms. Marchbanks ... this way to the treatment room; that's where we did your scan. You'll receive the radiation treatments in this room," she said, pointing to a doorway with a big lighted sign that read, CAUTION RADIATION IN USE.

My mouth went dry. I had mentally prepared myself for the other room; I was all set to go into the other room! This change in plans was unsettling to say the least. She walked ahead of me into the darkened room and as she stepped aside to let me pass, I froze. Staring back at me from the center of the room was a huge, ominous looking machine. The very sight of it crumbled what little nerve I had worked up and left me shaken and afraid.

"Ms. Marchbanks? Is everything okay?"

"No, actually. I've never seen this machine before; I thought we were going to the other room," I said as my stomach fluttered.

"Are you alright? Would you like for me to get the doctor?"

"No, I just wish I had known about this room before, so I could have prepared myself," I replied. My feet felt like they had been glued to the floor as I struggled to take a step forward toward the beast.

External Beam Radiation Machine — that's the official name of the mammoth piece of equipment, but to me it looked like something out of a science fiction horror movie and I didn't like it; I didn't like it at all. There were two other therapists in the room to assist with the procedure and at that moment all eyes were on me as I slowly walked toward the table and sat down.

The lead therapist approached me and said in a calm, friendly voice, "Just take your arms out of the sleeves and lie back. We won't uncover you until everything's set up." Therapist number two brought over the arm mold they had created for me and slid it under my head while a third therapist slid a bolster under my knees to support my back. They adjusted the position of my arms to fit the mold and then guided my hands toward a metal bar just above my outstretched arms. When all was said and done, the mental imagery of me lying on the table in that position, exposed and vulnerable, transported me back to medieval times and suddenly it was as if I were there and about to be tortured on the rack. It was all too much for me and I began to cry.

"Are you okay? Do you want us to get the doctor?" the lead therapist asked.

I shook my head no and she handed me a tissue with which to dry my eyes. I took a deep breath and said, "I'm okay; it's just all so surreal, you know? Let's just get this over with."

She pulled back the hospital gown exposing my right breast then located the tattoo dots, applied a clear round dot about the size of a quarter over them and then crossed through each one with a pink highlighter.

"You'll keep these tabs on for the duration. Don't even take them off when you shower, but if they happen to fall off, don't worry, we can replace them," she instructed.

When she had completed her task, she crossed the room to stand near a computer while the other two therapists moved into place on either side of the table. Beams of light shown like cross-hairs on my chest while coordinates numbers were called out by the lead therapist.

"Ninety-three, ninety-two point three, ninety-seven

point three, ninety-five point two," she announced. The therapist on my right raised or lowered the table by using a hydraulic foot pedal. The therapist to my left slid the sheet underneath me to the left or right simultaneously, rolling me until the beams of light and the tattoo dots were in perfect alignment. Together, they were a well orchestrated team.

"Everything looks perfect," the therapist to my right said then added, "It's very important that you hold this position until we finish the treatment; try to remain as still as possible until we tell you it's okay to move."

With that said they retreated to a control room a few feet away and watched me from behind a glass window.

"We'll still be able to see you and hear you, Ms. Marchbanks, so just call out if you need us, okay?"

"Okay," I replied and closed my eyes and began to pray.

The sound of the machine startled me as it awoke from its slumber. There were a series of mechanical movements and clicking noises and then a high pitched noise that sounded like a copy machine as it scans the paper. I kept my eyes closed the entire time and cringed as I waited for whatever was to come next.

"Okay! You can lower your arms and get dressed now," I heard the lead therapist announce as she walked back into the room. I had been holding onto the metal bar for dear life and in less than fifteen minutes the entire procedure from beginning to end was over. It took more time for me to drive there than it took to be treated, and what's more, I didn't feel a thing — no heat, no air, no pain, nothing.

They lowered the table back to its original position and helped me up.

"That's it, you're all done," she said. "And we'll go through the same procedure every day you come in, so no more surprises." she smiled.

I apologized for my earlier reaction and followed her out of the room and back across the hall to change. Two more women had arrived and were waiting patiently to be seen. Two more lives, two more families touched by cancer and I thought to myself, *sometimes your sisters are born and sometimes they are created by circumstance.*

Overflowing with emotion by the time I got dressed and to my car, all I could do was cry. *I can't do this, Lord! I'm just not strong enough. I can't do this by myself.* And just as He always does, he heard my cries and sent an angel to comfort me. My phone chimed with a text message from one of my spiritual sisters. *"Hey, Karrie! Just checking on you. I knew this was your first day of treatment and wanted you to know I'm praying for you. Call me if you need anything!"*

Through my tears I managed to text back a message thanking her for her prayers and told her I would call later. But later would come and go as I received call after call and text upon text from well wishers who wanted me to know they were praying for me. Their words of encouragement and heaven sent prayers held me up like crutches until I was able to speak to my Father about what had happened that day, as if He didn't already know.

That evening, before I went to bed, I put on my worship music and just listened for awhile before I began to pray. The words from the music removed the heaviness from my spirit and before I knew it, tears were streaming down my face and a sweet peace had washed over me, lifting me out of the depths of despair and placing me softly into the hands of Jesus. That mental image of the Lord carrying me in His hands and the juxtaposition of how big He is compared to me and my puny problems, gave me a new found strength, a power like I've never felt before and all the pain, all the fear, all the doubt had disappeared until all that was left was ... love.

The next day when I arrived at the office for treatment, I felt empowered! I walked in there like I owned it ... a stark contrast from the day before and the feeling was electric! For the first time since my diagnosis, I had a clear picture of what this trial was all about. It wasn't about me ... never was. No test ever is! The image God showed me of Him holding me in His hands was one of surrender. All He ever wants is for us to surrender our will for His and if we can do that, He'll carry us safely to our destiny. There would be no more tears of sorrow shed from my eyes, no more pleading, for now I was all about my Father's work and I was anxious to get started.

The first week went by without a hitch. The treatments were going well, my skin showed no signs of damage and I continued to work and exercise every day. The calendar they had given me on the first day now hung proudly on the refrigerator and I crossed off the days as they went by. Everyone in the office knew me, whether they wanted to or not. I took autographed copies of my book to the receptionists and made every effort to get to know the women who shared the waiting room with me. After a few days it was obvious who had the appointments before and

after yours, so I thought we might as well enjoy each other's company, and we did. These women had incredible stories to tell and I listened in amazement as they shared their testimonies with me.

One woman's story was similar to mine in that she had always lived a healthy, active lifestyle and then one day she finds out she has stage 3 lung cancer. She said she had been out playing tennis one day and noticed her breathing was labored. She rationalized it away as just being old and out of shape and made a mental note to herself to make more time to play. A couple of days later; however, she noticed that after climbing a flight of stairs she struggled to catch her breath. An appointment with her doctor confirmed the worst, and after surgery and a round of chemo she was here, undergoing radiation treatments. She told me she had been blindsided by the diagnosis as she had never smoked a day in her life. She was a single mom, her children were her life and even now she still found it difficult to come to grips with it all. We shared a hug that day and I prayed and asked God to send a blessing of strength and healing her way.

The therapist called my name and I rose from my seat to follow her. *Yea, though I walk through the valley of the shadow of death, I will fear no evil; for You are with me; Your rod and Your staff, they comfort me.* I boldly entered the treatment room and made conversation with the therapists as I approached the table to lie down. The shift in the atmosphere was palpable, and there was nothing the enemy could do about it. As soon as they were finished prepping me and the treatment began, I closed my eyes and started praising God. *Hallelujah! Hallelujah! You are worthy to be praised! Glory, glory, glory, you are worthy to be praised! Hineni, Lord! Hineni! I am here, Lord! Send me! Use me for your Glory! Thank you, Jesus, for your sacrifice; thank you for loving me and for never giving up on me. You are my strength, my joy, my love. I love you, Lord; I am here! Hallelujah!* I was so caught up in my praise that the time just flew by! When the therapist walked back into the room and told me I could sit up, I was almost annoyed at the interruption. I left the building that day transformed and glowing from the inside out.

Week two came and I had found my groove. I had a preferred parking space; I knew the information desk volunteers by name, had found the hospital café and became acquainted with yet another survivor in the waiting room. She was a young woman who was battling breast cancer. It was her first day of radiation treatment, although she had already been through a round of chemo. She had received a double mastectomy and shared with me how her mother was a breast cancer survivor of fifteen years. We never exchanged names; we didn't need to. The relationship we shared was beyond the superficial. Because of our circumstances we shared an understanding; we were soul sisters, and every day I looked forward to our random conversations about nothing and everything; solving the world's problems ten minutes at a time.

The therapist walked in and called my name. "Ms. Marchbanks, we're ready for you." Together, we walked back to the treatment room chatting about the rainy weather and how we were both ready for the weekend. By now I was a pro at positioning myself on the table and challenged myself to get it perfect every time. *Ninety-three, ninety-two point three, ninety-seven point three, ninety-five point two.* I had heard the numbers so many times I knew them by heart.

The machine started and just as I was about to close my eyes and begin to pray, a small voice whispered in my ear. *"No. Today, you're going to do this with your eyes open."* I acknowledged the Lord's presence, took a deep breath and watched as the arm of the machine swung into place. At the end of the arm was a big round disk — the head of the monster. It had bolts for eyes and appeared to be looking back at me as it hovered over my body. Its mouth was formed by the metal plates which opened and closed to direct the field of radiation. My body shuddered at the site, but my eyes held the monster's gaze and I began to pray. There were clicking sounds as the mouth adjusted to the proper size and then came a high pitched laser sound as the wave of radiation was sent like fire from a dragon's mouth into the left side of my breast. The machine held its position for a few seconds, and then moved up and over my body to the right and adjusted itself once again before emitting the last dose of radiation.

"You can bring your arms down; we're all done," the therapist announced as she walked back into the room. *I did it! I did it! Thank you, Jesus!* The smile on my face was confirmation that I had just slayed the beast, and in doing so, had replaced fear with strength. I left the room smiling from ear to ear.

Friday's were consultation days with Dr. Bobian, so I went to the exam room and waited for him to arrive. He entered the room with Kim, his nurse, following close behind. We exchanged greetings and then he took a seat on a stool and began to ask me a series of questions. "How are you feeling today? Your eyes look red; are you getting enough sleep? How's your appetite? Are you experiencing any skin issues like nipple soreness, burning, itching or feeling fatigued?" My answers came as quickly as his questions while the nurse stood by ready to take the doctor's orders if need be. He performed a quick breast examination to assess whether there were any visible signs of radiation damage like tanning, blistering or infection, and then listened to my lungs for signs of damage, which is also a potential risk when undergoing radiation treatment for breast cancer. The examination proved all was good and he even expressed his surprise that so far, my skin had remained unchanged. I told him I felt good and that I was still exercising five days a week.

"Just be careful," he said, "and listen to your body. If you're tired, rest. If you're sleepy, take a nap and make sure to eat even if you don't feel like it. Right now your body is in a constant state of healing and it needs all the energy it can get to perform that process. It's completely normal to experience some fatigue."

"I hear you, and I do rest. By the end of the day, I'm so ready to go to bed that I'm asleep as soon as my head hits the pillow! I haven't slept this good in years!" I replied, laughing.

After my visit with Dr. Bobian I went to the changing room and did a little victory dance in my stall. I'm sure the women sitting in the waiting room thought I was having a breakdown, but I didn't care; it was time to celebrate! I had just confronted the enemy, looked him straight in the eye and didn't even blink! Hallelujah!

By the end of the third week the skin on my right breast had started to tan, which was so weird and a little bit scary when you think about the how and why. A line of demarcation now separated the pale skin of my torso from the newly tanned skin of my breast and it looked as though I had a reverse bikini tan. The nipple had darkened and had become very sore, which made wearing a bra less than comfortable. By the end of the day, all I wanted to do was walk around topless. Underwire bras were out of the question and sports bras were too constricting, so after several failed attempts at trying to find a bra that didn't feel like sandpaper against the delicate skin, I chose to wear a simple, inexpensive nursing bra. The design was simple and the extra padding an added bonus.

"*To Bra or Not to Bra*" was the topic of conversation among the women in the waiting room one day and we laughed as some of them described the freedom they were experiencing from letting it all hang out. Obviously, I wasn't one of them and I laughed at the mental image of me and my *girls* bouncing freely down the street for the whole world to see.

I was excited when I went in for treatment that Friday; I had made two dozen of my famous, super soft almond sugar cookies and couldn't wait to share them in celebration of my three-week anniversary.

"Oh, my gosh; are these for us? Did you make them? They smell so good!" the receptionist said.

"Thank you and yes, I made them to celebrate my three-week milestone. I'm halfway done, can you believe it?"

"Wow, has it been that long?" she asked.

We chatted a little while longer and she assured me she would share the cookies with the other staff, that is, after she had put a few aside for herself.

Over the next three weeks the buildup of radiation began to take its toll; I was tired. Mornings came too quickly after sleepless nights from struggling to find a comfortable position. The damaged skin was now itching, fragile and sore. Things I had previously taken for granted like taking a shower or even dressing myself were now strategically planned out maneuvers. Even the seatbelt, created to save my life, was now a source of irritation and pain.

I stopped exercising after week five; I couldn't take the pain, but continued to work on a limited schedule. There were days when all I wanted to do was sleep and others when my body hurt so bad it brought me to tears. My ingrained sense of modesty eroded and I ditched the bra in favor of camisoles and loose fitting clothing for the remaining treatments.

By week six I was mentally and physically exhausted from trying to gracefully exist. The mask of fortitude that covered my face hid the torment that raged inside of me. On one hand I could finally see light at the end of the tunnel, but on the other hand the last eight treatments would prove to be the most difficult. The scar left behind from the surgery had started to keloid, and it was very sore and itched like crazy. Dr. Bobian prescribed a cortisone cream to help with the itching and attempt to reduce its size in conjunction with the next few treatments. The skin on my breast was so dark, it looked like it belonged to someone else, and I was in so much pain that it hurt to breathe. My faith swayed back and forth with each new day and started to unravel until it hung dangling by a single thread. *I trust you, Lord. I trust you! But I am so tired. Help me stay strong. Help me, Lord!*

That Friday, the end of week six, I woke with such energy I knew God had heard my prayers. There were only three treatments left and it was time to celebrate! I took my favorite dessert, an Italian wedding cake, to the staff that day to show my appreciation and to share with my sisters in the waiting room. They were thrilled!

"You told us you were going to celebrate at week six. We half expected you to walk in carrying balloons!" the receptionist said.

"Well, I hope you're not disappointed with cake,

'cause I can take it back!" I replied.

"No, ma'am! We accept all sweets!" she said.

Still laughing as I entered the waiting room, I announced to the women sitting there that I had brought cake to celebrate my six-week milestone and told them to make sure they let the nurses know if they wanted a piece before they left. The room erupted with cheers and clapping, which prompted the therapist to come investigate what all the commotion was about.

"You guys are way too happy. What's going on in here?" she asked jokingly.

"I brought cake!" I told her.

"Well, let's get this party started then!" she said while doing a little dance. "Just come on back when you're ready, Ms. Marchbanks."

I took a deep breath as I lay back on the table and assumed the position. *Ninety-three, ninety-two point three, ninety-seven point three, ninety-five point two.* This would be the last time I would hear those coordinates; next week they would be changed for the boost.

"I love your shoes, Ms. Marchbanks!" the therapist said as she pointed at the blue sequined flats that sparkled on my feet. "It's funny, you know; we never get to see a person's whole outfit … just the shoes."

"Thank you. I wore them on purpose today. I call them my happy shoes," I replied.

"And you have every reason to be happy; you're almost done!" she said.

I closed my eyes as the machine found its position over me and I began to praise God just as I had for the last thirty days. *Thank you, Lord, for your grace. Thank you, Lord, for your mercy. Thank you, Lord, for loving me in spite of who I am.*

Forgive me, Lord, my sins and cleanse my heart. Help me stay on the path to my destiny for you are my Lord and Savior. I bless your Holy name! All of you Lord, none of me! All of you, none of me! Hineni Lord, hineni! Glory, glory, glory! You are worthy to be praised!
The session ended, I met with Dr. Bobian, and then went home to sleep. Today was a good day.

The last three days of treatment were the worst in terms of how I felt and how my skin reacted. It was turning black under my arm and was starting to look like parchment paper. Every movement was painful and it felt as if it were on fire, no matter how much cream I applied.

The phone rang; it was a friend from church. I almost didn't take the call because I was just about to leave the house to go in for treatment.

"Hi, Brooke, how are you?" I said.

"I was calling you to ask the same thing," she said. Brooke had been through this routine a couple of years before. She had stage two breast cancer and had undergone chemo and radiation, so she knew the drill. During our conversation the topic of my skin came up.

"Why aren't you using shea butter?" She scolded.

"The doctor prescribed a cream; I've been using it three times a day," I replied.

"No, that stuff doesn't work! The best thing to heal your skin is shea butter. That's what I used when I went through it and I never had any problems. I'll bring you some."

Forty-five minutes later she met me in the hospital parking lot carrying a small container of organic, yellow shea butter.

"Call me tomorrow and let me know how your skin feels," she said. I thanked her, told her I would definitely call her and went on to my appointment.

Dr. Bobian had asked to meet with me before I changed to discuss the new treatment plan, so I sat in the exam room awaiting his arrival. The "*boost*," as he called it, meant that a higher dosage of radiation would be targeted at the surgical site where the cancer cells had been removed. The tissue in this much smaller area is where cancer is most likely to return, so having the boost helps reduce the chances of it coming back. My specific treatment plan would require three more days at the higher levels.

He went on to explain possible side effects and told me it was not uncommon for patients to develop scar tissue at the site or an infection from the boost and asked me to keep an eye on the area for any signs of redness.

"Do you have any questions?" he asked.

"Will it hurt?"

"You won't feel a thing, just like before."

Before he released me he checked the keloid for signs of improvement and thankfully it had indeed begun to smooth out.

When the machine locked into position it hovered directly over the top of me. The mouth opened and closed to fit the new coordinates and then emitted a beam of radiation about three inches in diameter around my surgical scar. The procedure went faster than before because of the smaller treatment area. *One down, two to go. Thank you, Lord, for giving me the strength to do this. I couldn't have done it without you. Your love lifts me up and I thank you for all the blessings you have given me and those I have yet to see. I praise your Holy name! All of you, Lord, none of me. All of you, none of me. In Jesus' name I pray, Amen.*

I was back in the changing room within minutes applying a thin layer of the shea butter over my right breast. To my surprise and delight, it felt like cool water dousing the flames of my irritated skin and I felt relief for the first time in weeks. *Thank you, Lord, for sending me another angel.*

The last two treatments of the boost were over before I knew it. My skin, although very damaged, was at least more comfortable since using the shea butter. Dr. Bobian said I was lucky; my skin had fared better than most patients he'd seen. *There's that word again — lucky. If they only knew.*

"I want you to watch out for signs of infection like fever, redness or warmth in the boost area, okay? The worst is over and from this day forward your body will begin restoring itself. You'll start to feel better and have more energy, but the radiation will continue to work inside the tissues for several more weeks. Try to stay out of the sun and keep your skin covered. And call us if you have any questions or concerns."

"I will. Is that it?" I asked.

"That's it for me, but stop at the nurse's station before you leave," he said.

I was taken aback by my feelings of ambivalence. During the entire course of this journey I felt as though everything were out of my control, like I was just supposed to be a good little girl and follow orders. And now, suddenly, they're telling me it's over, get on with your life, you're free to go! Free to go do what? So I made light of the situation and said, "Okay. Thank you, Dr. Bobian; it was a pleasure getting to know you, but I hope I never see you again! Don't even say hello if you see me on the street. We are not friends."

"Yeah, I get that a lot," he said with a smile and we shook each other's hand before he and the nurse left the room.

After changing clothes I stopped at the nurse's station for what I assumed were discharge papers, but I couldn't have been more wrong.

"Hi, Kate; Dr. Bobian said you needed to see me?"

"Yes! Before we let you go I want you to choose a stone from this vase."

Oh! I thought to myself, *how cool! I get to take one of these home as a memento.* So I reached down into the pile and sifted through the colored glass until I found one that would look good with my home décor. It was a brown glass pebble with blue and white swirls running through it. I showed it to Kate.

"Great! Now come with me," she said, and we walked through the door leading to the reception area where we were immediately joined by the other members of my patient care team. They stood in front of me with smiles on their faces and my curiosity piqued.

Kate, acting as leader, began the ceremony with, "All of us at LCI Radiation Therapy Center want to congratulate you for getting through these treatments!" And everyone began to clap. She went on to say, "And, we want to say thank you for choosing us to journey with you as you battle your cancer. We hope we took excellent care of you, supported you and encouraged you during your treatments. And we'd like to say thank you, for the very special gift that you have given to each one of us — the gift of yourself! You brought us happiness every day with your laughter, your smile, and those delicious cookies!"

"Yes, and I'm going to need the recipe before you leave!" the receptionist said, and the entire group laughed.

Kate continued by saying, "We had you select a stone because we want to mark this special day by remembering you and this journey you have been on." Then she grabbed a vase filled with similar stones from a team member standing nearby.

"We keep this vase of stones as a reminder of you and how precious your life is. So, if you don't mind, we would like to have the stone you have chosen, too!" And she held out the vase in front of her. Her words struck my heart and my eyes began to sting as I gently lowered my pebble into the vase and let it rest on top of the others. I remembered seeing that vase on my first day and at the time had thought it was a cute desk top accessory. But now, knowing the significance of the pebbles and all the lives they represented brought tears to my eyes. I would never know the men and women who came before me, or those who would come after me for that matter, but here we remained – a testament that although our lives had been touched by cancer, the Lord's grace and mercy had given each of us the strength to make through to a brighter day.

"You guys are so amazing and thank you for all you've done. This is so unexpected! I can't begin to tell you how much this means to me," I said as I wiped the tears from my eyes. "But, I'm going to tell you just like I told Dr. Bobian; I hope we *never* see each other again!"

The ceremony ended, just as it should, with laugher and hugs as we said our goodbyes. I will never forget that day; it was officially the first day of the rest of my life, and the number one thing on my to-do list — sleep!

The drive home was exhausting as the events of the day had left me physically and emotionally drained. A colorful montage of all that had happened played in my head as I tried desperately to find a comfortable position on the sofa to take a nap, but sleep would have to wait. My phone chimed with a new text message from a friend.

"Why didn't you tell me about the book?" she asked.

I don't know what you're talking about, but I'll bite. "What book?" I replied.

"Your book! Sweet Tea and Cornbread!" she answered.

"What about it?"

"It was nominated for an award!"

"What?"

"Check out this link!" she urged.

I adjusted the pillows so I could sit up and clicked the link in the message. The page opened up and the header read *2013 African American Literary Awards*. I scrolled down to the bottom of the page, but didn't see anything that pertained to me or my book, so I called her.

"Okay, so what are you talking about, I don't see anything."

"Are you on the site? Click on the nominee link and scroll down to the bottom. Do you see it?"

I followed her instructions and there it was, right on the page in front of me — my name and the title of my book!

"Oh, my gosh! How did this happen? How did you find out? I didn't even know such an award even existed!"

I listened intently as she explained the series of events that led up to her texting the good news. I couldn't believe it! My book, my little book had been nominated for an award. But what's more than that, the news of the nomination came on my last day of treatment. Thirty-three days had passed and it was as if the Lord had just said, "Well done, my good and faithful servant." And in His perfect timing, I knew I had just received my victory! But that wasn't the end.

I wish I could tell you that my book won the award, but it didn't. I wish I could tell you I was all right with that, but I wasn't. I sat at the table that night, in that grand room, hair done, nails done, in the most expensive piece of clothing I had ever owned, waiting anxiously for them to announce the winner of my category.

"And the award goes to…" I turned toward my daughter so I could watch her reaction when they called my name and then quickly back to the presenter when the name she announced sounded nothing like mine. *You've got to be kidding me! There must be a mistake. I wrote a speech, I bought a dress! I came to New York to receive my victory…That's my award!* Now, don't get me wrong, there was no pity party! But I am only human, and for that brief moment it was all about *me!* It wasn't a question of feeling blessed or not. I knew I was blessed simply because I was alive and sitting there, but at the time that wasn't enough. I wanted the prize, the reward, that thing that I could hold in my hand and show the world — the *proof* that my faith was enough.

I came home from New York with stories to tell, but no tangible victory, and over the next few weeks I began to question what the last six months had all been about if not for that moment. The Lord gave me time, just as He always does, to come to my own conclusions, and when He decided I was making more of a mess of things than need be, I got a phone call from Pastor John.

"Hi, Pastor John," I said as I drove the car out of the hospital's parking garage.

"Hi, daughter, how are you? How's everything going?"

"Good, actually and thanks for asking. I just came from a follow-up appointment with the surgeon and she said everything looks good."

"That is awesome!" he replied.

"It's funny that you called at this time because I've had a lot on my mind lately."

"Like what?" he asked.

"Well, you know, the awards show for one thing. I really thought I was going to win. I just knew that God had given me my victory. To actually win the award would have been the icing on the cake! And now that I'm solidly on the road to recovery with this whole cancer thing, I hate to say it, Pastor John, but I almost feel unworthy of the term breast cancer survivor."

"Why would you say that?" he asked.

"Because … as traumatic and difficult as this whole ordeal was, there are so many women out there who have survived much worse. To be honest, I guess I don't feel like I suffered enough to earn the term survivor. I mean, I didn't have chemo, my body is still intact; to look at me you would never even know I had cancer."

"And why do you think that is?" he asked. His response surprised me.

"What do you mean?" I questioned.

"Well, first of all, don't down play all that you've just been through. You are a survivor in every sense of the word. And maybe the outcome of your diagnosis and the ease with which you experienced it has less to do with you and everything to do with your relationship with God."

"What do you mean?" I asked again.

"Wasn't it you who told me that while going through this trial you never stopped praising Him?"

"Yes."

"Well, perhaps you need to look again. You're not seeing the big picture. You focused in on one thing — the reward, but maybe God had something else in mind. Maybe he took you through this trial so that He could use you to share your testimony with other women. For, just like gold that can only be refined and shaped by fire to bring it to its purest form and usefulness, you, my dear, have just been through the fire and I think there's a story to be told."

His words hit me like a ton of bricks and a shiver ran icily up my spine. "Whoa, Pastor John! I've never thought about it like that."

"Then, perhaps, it's time you did."

My Testimony

To say that breast cancer changed my life would be an understatement, because it changed so much more than that. My very existence has been altered in ways I could never have imagined and now, as I look back a year later, I can't believe how far I've come physically and the growth I've experienced spiritually. My journey was hard, and there were days when I felt like I wouldn't make it. Yet, when you're in the midst of a battle, fighting for your life, the last thing on your mind is surrender. Well, what I've learned from what has been my toughest fight yet is that as Christians, our most powerful weapon in any battle we're faced with is precisely that — surrender.

As we are placed over the heat of testing, trials and tribulations, we are quick to decide that the intensity of the fire is too much for us to withstand and think that there is no way we will ever make it through. We doubt whether we are strong enough or fear that God isn't big enough. Being afraid is a natural part of human nature, while surrender is a supernatural act of faith. You've read my story. You know how I struggled with fear and doubt, and while I'm not proud of my moments of weakness, with each new test that came my way I was able to find the strength to let go of my fear and hold on to my faith long enough to get through. So, if you think my story is about my battle with breast cancer, you've missed the point. Breast cancer was only the catalyst that caused the surrender of my will for God's, and thus, allows me to testify to how something so devastating, so traumatic, so bad can be covered in grace and turned around for good. My testimony is about how I was able to see the good in cancer.

My first test of faith came when I listened to that still, small voice whispering in my ear; it told me to schedule a mammogram. I might not be here today had I remained stubborn and resolved to my opinion that because I was in good health, having a yearly mammogram was a waste of time. That seemingly simple act of surrendering my will for His changed my life. And I've learned that so often we miss God's blessing because we've lost our ability to hear the little things He is trying to tell us.

Moreover, the discovery of my breast cancer ushered in the next test of faith — surrendering my fear for His wisdom. I am not a doctor; I don't even play one on TV, so there was nothing I could do that I hadn't already done to keep cancer out of my body or to make it go away, except pray. Now, don't get me wrong; it wasn't easy! And the only way I could do it was to take myself out of the equation and trust that, *"All things work together for good to those who love God, to those who are called according to His purpose." Romans 8:28(KJV).* Making the decision to undergo surgery and then radiation therapy took a lot of faith and surrender — faith that I had the right team of caregivers, faith that I would have the money to pay the medical bills, and faith that I would survive at all! It would have been easy for me to project my fear onto the prognosis and worry myself into a state of depression. But I faithfully believed that if I just held on, God had something greater for me. What the Lord has showed me is this: If we will only surrender and let Him carry us through, tests and trials produce glory in us when we walk in faith. The fight is not over until God says it's over. So don't let go, don't give in! The Lord is on your side!

It's so easy for us to focus our attention and efforts on the problem at hand, but hopefully, not so much so that we end up creating a bigger problem. So remember, with every new challenge comes an opportunity to be blessed. Had I not surrendered and allowed God to use me, I would have never come to know all the wonderful women who sat with me in that waiting room. I wouldn't have cared about what they were going through, it wouldn't have bothered me when one of them didn't show up the next day and I surely wouldn't have been baking cookies and cakes! The challenge before me was to see past my pain; the opportunity was to share the Word of God and be a blessing to others and I'm so glad I didn't miss it!

Receiving word about the nomination of my book for an award on the last day of my radiation treatments was huge! It was just the reward I had been waiting for. Surely, the Lord had witnessed my faith and had found me worthy. But while I prepped and prepared to receive the coveted prize, the true blessing passed right over my head. When we covet things, even our own lives, we forget who we belong to. But when we let go of *things* and surrender to His will for our lives, the reward is already ours. It wasn't the Lord's intention for me to receive that award; His plan was for me to draw closer to Him so that he could use me for His glory. The challenge, breast cancer, brought about the opportunity, surrender, and I am more blessed now than I've ever been because of it.

The human drive to succeed is formidable all by itself. Couple that with the Holy Spirit and miracles abound! Though we often question God as to why we are going through challenges, we soon come to find that God is blessing us with the very thing we thought was the curse.

My prayer is that you and your loved ones live long and healthy lives, free from tests and trials, but in the event you must face adversity, I pray you will remember me and my story of surrender, and faithfully receive the blessing God has waiting just for you.

Breast Cancer Facts

- Yearly mammograms are recommended starting at age 40
- Clinical breast exam (CBE) about every 3 years for women in their 20s and 30s and every year for women 40 and over About 1 in 8 U.S. women (just over 12%) will develop invasive breast cancer over the course of her lifetime.
- Breast cancer survival rates go up when it's caught early. Don't miss your yearly mammogram!
- A woman's risk of breast cancer approximately doubles if she has a first-degree relative (mother, sister, daughter) who has been diagnosed with breast cancer. About 15% of women who get breast cancer have a family member diagnosed with it.
- More African American women die from treatable breast cancers than other races because they are in poorer health to begin with. i.e, high blood pressure, high cholesterol, heart disease, diabetes, obesity. (Most chronic diseases are preventable with healthy eating and exercise.)
- About 85% of breast cancers occur in women who have no family history of breast cancer. The most significant risk factors for breast cancer are gender (being a woman) and age (growing older).
- Do a monthly breast self-exam and report any changes to your doctor immediately.
- The CDC's National Breast and Cervical Cancer Early Detection Program (NBCCEDP) provides breast and cervical cancer screenings and diagnostic services to low-income, uninsured, and underinsured women across the U.S. www.cdc.gov/cancer/nbccedp/screenings.htm

Resources

Financial Assistance for Cancer Patients

- Managecancer.org
- Giveforward.com
- Knowcancer.com

Breast Cancer Awareness Websites

- National Comprehensive Cancer Network (NCCN): www.nccn.org
- National Breast Cancer Foundation: www.nationalbreastcancer.org
- Susan G. Komen Foundation: ww5.komen.org
- American Cancer Society (ACS): www.cancer.org
- American Society of Clinical Oncology (ASCO): www.asco.org
- National Cancer Institute (NCI): www.cancer.gov
- BreastCancer.org
- BreastCancerSociety.org
- BreastCancerAwareness.com

About the Author

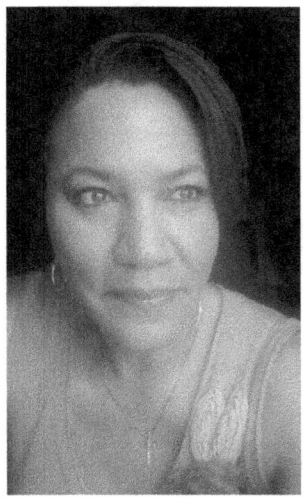

Karrie Marchbanks is a mother, entrepreneur, mentor, award-nominated author and breast cancer thriver! *Thirty-Three Days of Praise* is the second book to be penned by the author. Her first book *Sweet Tea and Cornbread: Inspiring, Motivating and Empowering Black Women to Take Back Their Bodies and Live a Healthier Lifestyle* was published in 2012 and nominated for a 2013 African American Literary Award.

When she's not championing the issues of women's health in America through speaking engagements, interviews, fundraisers and social media she enjoys traveling and crossing off items on her ever shrinking bucket list. Karrie currently resides in North Carolina.

www.ingramcontent.com/pod-product-compliance
Lightning Source LLC
Chambersburg PA
CBHW070202290526
45789CB00002B/877